Health and Medicine in Ancient Egypt

Magic and science

Paula Alexandra da Silva Veiga

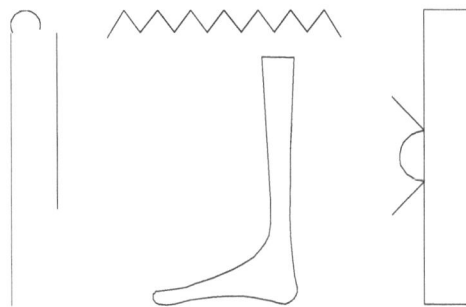

BAR International Series 1967
2009

Published in 2016 by
BAR Publishing, Oxford

BAR International Series 1967

Health and Medicine in Ancient Egypt

ISBN 978 1 4073 0500 4

BAR Publishing is the trading name of British Archaeological Reports (Oxford) Ltd.
British Archaeological Reports was first incorporated in 1974 to publish the BAR
Series, International and British. In 1992 Hadrian Books Ltd became part of the BAR
group. This volume was originally published by Archaeopress in conjunction with
British Archaeological Reports (Oxford) Ltd / Hadrian Books Ltd, the Series principal
publisher, in 2009. This present volume is published by BAR Publishing, 2016.

Printed in England

BAR
PUBLISHING

BAR titles are available from:

BAR Publishing
122 Banbury Rd, Oxford, OX2 7BP, UK
EMAIL   info@barpublishing.com
PHONE   +44 (0)1865 310431
FAX   +44 (0)1865 316916
www.barpublishing.com

Contents

" (…)
The hairs in my head are the same as the ones from the goddess Nun.
My face is the Solar disc of Ra.
The strength of the goddess Hathor lives in my eyes.
The soul of Upuaut[1] echoes inside my ears.
Inside my nose the forces of the god Khenti-Khas are alive.
My two lips are the lips of Anupu.[2]
My teeth are the teeth of Serket.
My neck is the neck of the goddess Isis.
My two hands are the hands of the powerful lord of Djedu.[3]
It is Neit, the sovereign of Sais that lives in my two arms.
My backbone is the backbone of Seth.
My phallus is the phallus of Osiris.
My flesh is the flesh of the Lords of Kher-Aha.
My chest is the Lord of the Terrors.
My womb and my back are those of the goddess Sekhmet.
The forces of the Eye of Horus dwell in my buttocks.
My legs are the legs of Nut.
My feet are the feet of Ptah.
My fingers are the fingers Of the Double Divine Falcon that lives forever.
In truth! There is no one member in my body that is not hosted by a divinity.
As for Thoth, he protects all my body.
As Ra, I renew myself everyday."[4]

---

[1] Or Wepwawet.
[2] Or Anubis.
[3] Or Osiris.
[4] Chapter 42 from The Book of the Dead, translated from the Portuguese, Sales, 1999: 419.

Introduction

Health was a constant concern in life and even the deceased needed extra care so that they would be at their prime when enclosed in the sarcophagus; and in the possession of magical 'weapons' so that when they reached the Afterlife, they would be in complete possession of all their physical abilities. Medicine in ancient Egypt was trying to restrain all malefic beings from action and to preserve the well-being of the individual. Thus the initial statement that magic and science were as one, a sole concept, was represented by

heka.

Through this work, all descriptions and conceptions observed in the existing legacy of ancient Egypt will lead to conclusions that attest this unique duality.

After careful observation, this work was divided into Chapters, because this format complies with the interconnection of the studied themes; investigating the Egyptian legacy and comparing it with multiple present examples, as part of the pathological patterns in Egypt did not change much when referring to endemic diseases.

There are four Chapters: Chapter 1: Sources of Information; Medical and Magical Papyri; Chapter 2:

Heka – "the art of the magical written word"; Chapter 3: Pathological types; Chapter 4: Medical-magical prescriptions and their ingredients; this list is a description that contemplates from the global perspective to details, revealing all, from general existing sources to particular ingredients used in prescriptions.

Chapter 1 (Sources of Information; Medical and Magical Papyri) briefly lists pertinent sources of information for the study of medical-magical practices in ancient Egypt. This includes some sources not quoted in this work, but nevertheless essential to this research, analysis and conclusive thinking. These are, Egyptian papyri, written in different languages, ostraca with medical-magical characteristics, skeletons and mummified human remains, art depictions, foreign travellers' diaries, general literature where pathologies are mentioned (personal letters), food habits, seasons of famine and abundance caused by war or natural catastrophes such as the yearly flood. The reference to the origin of the word *mummia* is made and also to the "mummy powder" used as medicine. Some ancient Egyptian words are listed which either relate to health and body parts, or mummification, just as examples. Further, the mummification procedures are summarised according to classical authors and their ideas of ancient Egypt regarding the human body. The chapter ends with some cases of analyzed Egyptian mummies, referring to the techniques used and results concluded. A table lists known cases.

In the second chapter (Chapter 2: *Heka* – "the art of the magical written word"), an analysis is made of how the ancient Egyptians considered magic, both in life, after death, in the afterlife, its relation to the human body, magical 'performances' and the desired effects. Also discussed is the 'job' and its application by priests, exorcists, doctors-magicians, the active practitioners of magic (those who produced medical prescriptions and applied them), how the medical diagnosis was made. In addition a table illustrating medical specialties is shown; some ancient Egyptian words are listed as related to human body parts and mummification, a question is posed about *per-ankh*, a hospital-school(?) and also a reference is made to medical instruments. Next comes a sub-chapter on written magic, spells and gods relating to magic and personal performances. Another sub-chapter lists different amulets and their importance; it also mentions some words used in personal protection, including human substances used as ingredients in magical prescriptions with medical intent.

In the third chapter (Chapter 3: Pathological types), some pathologies are discussed; the ones we can relate to ancient Egyptian society as to have existed mentioning treatments, when known.

In the fourth chapter (Chapter 4: Medical-magical prescriptions and their ingredients), the ancient Egyptian pharmacopoeia is discussed in more detail, identifying the type of ingredients used in prescriptions in vegetable, mineral and animal items, giving examples.

The conclusions are clear; magic and medicine did not exist as separate entities and were not distinct from each other. In ancient Egypt, the state of well-being was achieved by bringing together a mix of prophylactic actions (generally denominated as magic by modern Western civilizations), and medical treatments with a probable scientific basis.

1. State of the art

In researching health and medical practices in ancient Egypt we approach several aspects of life in Egypt, archaeology, religion,[5] as well as spoken and written languages in social daily life. This approach, based on data that represents probable copies of ancient written legacy does not allow for chronologically precise religious-magical-medical practices in ancient Egypt.

This work is, therefore, based on the known sources of information and concluding without exact dates.

For example, there is some doubt regarding some of the available data, such as the information given to us by Saint Clement of Alexandria, born *Titus Flavius Clemens*, (c.150 - 211/216)[6] on the possibility of the

existence of scientific encyclopaedias, such as 42 volumes originally thought to have been written by Thoth, six of them about medicine, from the Old Kingdom.[7] This information is just that: an hypothesis. Based on this the introduction is built, and here you can read, intellectually analyze or even risk to state that, these books described all the observation, diagnosis and therapeutics involved in ancient Egyptian science. These volumes would be, according to Clement of Alexandria, describing the constitution of the human body, its pathologies, organs, general medical prescriptions, eye treatments, and treatments for womens' diseases. It is also important to mention those who studied at Alexandria in Greco-Roman times as well as those practices in the Coptic and Arabic Periods. It would have been in this important Egyptian city in Hellenistic times that the reminiscences of pharaonic times influenced the knowledge and practices.

With that in mind, we can still repeat what was done at that time and have ideas about how some present popular beliefs go back to Pre-Dynastic times, even though we have no direct written or iconographic evidence of it from so long ago in Egypt. However, we do have oral tradition and many of the myths still reflect intertwined cosmogonies; gods that have several abilities and competences which are sometimes melt into syncretic ones. In the Ptolemaic period (c. 305-30 BC) and also in Greco Roman (30 BC to AD 395), Byzantine (middle 4th century to 642) or even Arabic periods these medical-magical practices of ancient Egypt persisted, with some adaptations. This can be seen from the iconography; there is continuous visual change throughout these periods and also in the amulets that combine divinities from different religious beliefs[8] and these are discussed in Chapter 2: *Heka* – "the art of the magical written word").

Also of importance for our research are the diaries of travellers to Egypt since Classical times (doctors in Alexandria), letters sent from and to other countries such as Assyria, Palestine and Mesopotamia (not used for this work but nevertheless important to mention and to include as sources of information) and Arabs and Europeans established in Egypt in the 18th (Napoleon's expedition), 19th and 20th centuries.

It is from the Nile that most of the information is taken for the study of the health and personal hygiene of the ancient Egyptians, as they survived thanks to this river.

---

[5] Lenoir, 2005 : 4-6.
[6] Titus Flavius Clemens, first known theologian from the Christian Church of Alexandria. In his *Stromata*, or *Miscellania*, Book I, chapter

XVI, this author states, regarding medicine in ancient Egypt that: "and they say that Phoenician and Syrian invented the letters first; and that Ápis, an aboriginal inhabitant of Egypt, invented the healing art before Io (God, *yawveh* in Hebrew; *Iao* in Greek) arrived in Egypt. But then they say that Asclepius improved the art"
http://www.ccel.org/ccel/schaff/anf02.toc.html
[7] London
[8] Veiga, Paula, 2008, *Preliminary Study of an Unusual Graeco-Roman Magical Gem (MNA E540) in the National Museum of Archaeology in Lisbon, Portugal*, CRE VIII, Kenneth Griffin (ed.) (with collaboration with Meg Gundlach), Oxbow Books, Oxford, p.141-150.

Herodotus was the one who said that (5th century BC): "Egypt was the gift of the Nile".

Every year the rivers' flood brought life and prosperity, starting mid-July and ending mid September, with the deposit of the black land onshore, Kemet (the black land refers to the dark colour of the nutrient rich water which was visible as it settled on the Nile shores), and as an opposition to Desheret (the red land as a comparison to the scorching sands of the desert). In today's Egypt the endemic diseases are the same and parasitical ones, affecting the eyes and the digestive tract, are caused by Nile water infections as a result of bacterial activity.

Nile, the river, *iteru*, ⟨hieroglyphs⟩, *itrw*, was the chain of life but also the bearer of disease, as contaminated waters infected food as it was cooked and cleaned and used as drinking water (as still today in rural Egypt). Water was seen as a purifying element but this might only apply in truth to the sacred lakes and even those might also be contaminated by animals and insects. The sacred lakes were kept so that priests, pilgrims and the sick could bathe and cleanse themselves from impurities, both physical and spiritual.

Running Nile waters and its channels were subjected to animal and human defecation, sand deposit, wood and stone debris deposit (from construction works), rotten carcasses of animals and also decomposing plants from sun action, insect eggs and larvae and other infectious elements brought by the flood and manual labour. As the flood levels varied each year, so these populations had more abundance or could experience famines if the waters did not rise high enough to plant seeds, This, of course was reflected in the general populations' state of health. There were 3 seasons:

Akhet, flood[9]   Peret, water descent[10]   Chemu, harvest[11]

⟨hieroglyphs⟩   ⟨hieroglyphs⟩   ⟨hieroglyphs⟩
3ht   *prt*   *šmw*

There is literature about Great famines and abundant years as well.

Starting our trip in the 4th century, in Alexandria, autopsies[12] and body dissection were already being made, as Aretaeus of Cappadocia states.[13] Among several descriptions we can mention Herodotus, Book II, *Histories*, published around 430 BC or 424 BC, also Diodorus Siculus, who's visit to Egypt can be dated by the 180th Olympics (60 to 56 BC); Strabo, a geographer

who visited Egypt during the reign of Augustus (27 BC-14 AD), and Gaius Plinius Secundus, (23-79 AD), known as Pliny the Elder, who wrote the *Naturalis Historia*, where he revealed many phytotherapeutical procedures used in Egypt. This author seemed to have a great knowledge of human physiognomy and medicine in general.

Jumping to a more recent period of Egyptian History in the medical point of view, we our journey from the moment when Napoleon brought Egypt to the world.

In 1798 Bonaparte brought thousands of men with him to Egypt, among them were soldiers, men from sciences, letters and arts and this expedition resulted in the publication of the *Description de l'Égypte*[14] in 37 volumes, published in Paris shortly after his return from the trip. It was during this expedition of 35,000 soldiers, 167 'wise men' and some hundred civilians, that the Rosetta Stone was discovered and this allowed another Frenchman, Jean François Champollion (1790-1832) to decipher the writing of ancient Egypt some years later.

Denon[15] also took part in this expedition of 1798 participating in this adventure, we might say, as the first 'Egyptologist'.[16] "All my life I wished for this trip to Egypt...", he says at the beginning of his diary. "Denon is the first European to describe, examine, draw, measure and comment on the monuments of pharaonic Egypt and by so, giving them the right to eternity."[17] He says "...I was going to unveil a new country..." Regarding healthcare in Egypt, Denon describes some situations that may not be far from ancient Egypt: "it was so hot that the Sun burned my feet through the shoes;[18] "The solstice sun burned our blood...";[19] "caused bleedings in the nose, giving us painful exaltations that covered all body parts randomly, dried and hardened the skin and made breathing very difficult. The sunrays, the main or even the sole cause of our evils, made us feel in all the pores a kind of sting, very similar to the ones produced by syphilis (would he have suffered from this disease?), that become unbearable when, to lie down, it is necessary to lie down over all these painful spots."[20]

Even the reference to the symbol of medicine[21] was made by Denon after these observations: "...we have out it along a bat and it became the goddess of health. The Egyptians connected two of them around a globe, so it would maybe represent the balance of the world system."[22] Describing the relationship between magic and

---

[9] Faulkner, 2006: 4.
[10] Faulkner, 2006: 90.
[11] Faulkner, 2006: 267.
[12] Autopsy: coming from the Greek root meaning "to see for one's self." The first documented human dissection was made by Herophilus. He dissected more than 600 cadavers of condemned criminals (Malomo, 2006).
[13] Calne, 2000: 60.

[14] Digital version available online at: http://*descegy.bibalex.org/*
[15] 1747-1825.
[16] Denon, 2004: 24.
[17] Denon, 2004: 19 (introduction).
[18] Denon, 2004: 226.
[19] Denon, 2004: 200.
[20] Denon, 2004: 249.
[21] The Rod of Asclepius, a single snake entwined around a stick. Caduceus used mainly in pharmaceutical themes: two snakes around a stick; Wilcox and Whitham, 2003, 138: 673-677.
[22] Denon, 2004:120.

medicine in Egypt, Denon says that "They think that the spiritual impoverished people, when dead, have powers and influence; one is the Father of Light and cures the evil from the eyes. Another is the Father of the generation and presides all births, etc.", and, further, regarding a magical tree: "I have found hair tied with nails, teeth, small bags of leather, little standards and close to tombs, from isolated stones, a place in the shape of a saddle under which there was a thick lamp. Hair was nailed by women to pin down the inconsistency of their husbands. The teeth belonged to adults that consecrated them to implore the return of the latter."[23] There is even a description of the diseases that struck the human forces of this expedition: "The heat of the days, the freshness of nights in that season afflicted the army with a large number of ophthalmia: this disease is avoidable when large walks or fatigue are followed by camping in which the humidity in the air replicates perspiration, these produces swellings that attack the eyes or the internal organs."[24]

The heat was a constant disturbance, as Denon states: "We are suddenly surprised with a heart pain and no help can prevent the fainting that follows within which the unhappy struck collapses."[25] The existence of the *khamsin*, an annual southwest strong Saharan wind that swipes across Egyptian lands for around fifty days (as its name in Arabic says) between April and June, did not go without notice to the participants of this expedition. It was called a hurricane by Denon: "the colors of the horizon change, the animals wander about the fields, in the river the water grows (...) agitating the bottom of the river under the feet. A Great amount of dust in the air tears out the eyes clouded by the arisen dust. Lightning can be seen, it rains a lot and the plague of the desert grasshopper[26] appears. The Nile course seems to become straighter and its waters are muddy and stinky, the winds change in direction and compress the lungs at such velocity."[27]

As a curiosity there is a reference to the water of the Wadi el-Ambagi in Qosseir at the Red Sea coast that, being mineral water in a sterile soil, would give sobriety to the local inhabitants and this meant a low level of diseases as no doctor was recorded at that place.[28] Wilkinson,[29] in 1847, describes both Egyptian landscapes and Pharaonic legacy, that there are few diseases there: "The diseases in Egypt are few."[30] He says that the fevers

are rare, except in the Mediterranean coast and those foreigners, (non-Egyptian people) who complain about dysentery and ophthalmia. Furthermore, he presents medical prescriptions to take and suggests how to protect the eyes and protect yourself from the climate, speaks of the 'plague', that may refer to an infectious disease (malaria), and he advises on the evacuation to Upper Egypt as "...it never goes above Osioót" (Assiut) or to stay in quarantine, if you are in Lower Egypt.

According to another Frenchman, Desgenettes, (1762-1837), Chief-Physician of Napoleon's army, who set up new and strict hygiene and prophylactic practices when commissioned to Egypt, such as the cleaning of clothing, places and the control of food hygiene, "the extreme sobriety of the Egyptians (...) is a contribution for the well-being and to extend the existence in this country, as well as the air and the water (...), diseases that afflict like plagues, dysentery and chicken pox. The most common, affecting one third of the population [Cairo] is a kind of disease of the eye; no other town has so many blind people. Each four or five years, the plague [cholera] escalates in Cairo in a violent way. (...)". This doctor observed cases of small pox, scurvy, conjunctivitis and dysentery.[31]

With the discovery and further sale of magical and medical papyri, the majority of them from the 19th century, there are Egyptologists interested in decoding the medical prescriptions, their ingredients and the spells/prayers that were recited over the treatments to the patient. In the 19th century some names are already referenced as important to the study of medicine in ancient Egypt. They were mainly French doctors commissioned in Egypt by French rulers and were innovating the health system implanted in the Egyptian population and trying to fight endemic diseases. This curiosity for ancient Egyptian medicine naturally developed in them, as its roots are still visible in contemporary popular beliefs.

Egypt was visited by Antoine Barthelemy Clot[32] (1793-1868), a French doctor known as Clot Bei, born in Grenoble, and educated at Montpellier. After practicing for some time at Marseille he was promoted to Chief Surgeon by Muhammad Ali, viceroy of Egypt. In Abuzabel, near Cairo, Antoine Barthelemy Clot founded a hospital and schools to teach medicine, and also, with religious opposition by the Egyptians themselves, the study of anatomy by dissection of cadavers. In 1832

---

[23] Denon, 2004:126.
[24] Denon, 2004:130.
[25] Denon, 2004: 254.
[26] Desert locust, *Schistocera gregaria*
[27] Adapted from Denon, 2004: 236, 246.
[28] Denon, 2004: 242.
[29] Handbook for Travellers in Egypt, 1847, Sir John Gardner Wilkinson (1797–1875)
[30] The diseases of Egypt are few. Fevers are very rare, except around Alexandria, Damietta, and other places on the coast; and almost the only complaints to which strangers are subject to inland are diarrhœa, dysentery, and ophthalmia. The following is a good mode of treatment for diarrhœa or even for the beginning of suspected dysentery. Wilkinson, 1847: I, c.

---

http://scholarship.rice.edu/jsp/xml/1911/9190/1095/WilEgyp.tei-timea.html (pages 6-7 in the paper edition).
[31] http://www.medarus.org/Medecins/MedecinsTextes/desgenettes.html
[32] Clot Bei (Antoine Barthelemy Clot), French surgeon, recruited by Muhammad Ali. He established a medical school, and launched the basis of the Egyptian Public Health Service. His collection of Egyptian items was sold to the council of Marseille, France, http://weekly.ahram.org.eg/2005/766/sc3.htm; some of his work, *Relation des épidémies de cholera qui ont régné de l'Heggaz, a Suez, et en Egypte* (1832), *De La Peste observe en Egypte* (1840), *Aperçu général sur l'Egypte*, 2 vols. (1840).

Muhammad Ali proclaimed him Bei, an important title, without him having to convert to Islamic religion; and in 1836 he was promoted to general and chief of the medical board in Egypt. In 1849 he returned to Marseille, but went back to Egypt in 1856, and he died in 1868.

In the development of paleopathology in the 20th century some distinguished names were pioneers in mummies' autopsies, as Sir Marc Armand Ruffer, professor of Bacteriology in Cairo Medical School, said himself "the science of disease demonstrated in human and animal remains is found in ancient tissue".[33]

Also the Belgian Frans Jonckheere (1903-1956), from Brussels, a surgeon and a gynecologist, counted 82 doctors by name in the *Description*, undertook extensive research on the diseases from ancient Egypt.[34]

In Egyptology, the branches of study are diverse, from daily life to ancient Egyptian practices regarding hygiene, food and health and these studies start to become relevant in some Egyptologists' research, but only at the end of the 20th century. Until the 1920's and 1930's of this century, literature and linguistics were the main themes in Egyptology, which came into existence after Champollion deciphered the hieroglyphics in 1822. In the following decades of the 20th century, 50s, 60s and 70s, religion was the dominant theme in published work, although there have been constant excavations in Egypt since the 19th century and the antiquity market brought many pieces to the Museums. However, what would have contributed mostly to the advance of biomedical Egyptology was the evolution of techniques, more precise thus enabling surprising results.

2. The investigation of pathology patterns through mummified human remains and art depictions from ancient Egypt

"The lacuna is the most dynamic factor in the study of ancient inscriptions. Here everything is to be found"[35]

Bearing in mind that, in bone analysis, many diseases do not last long enough to leave a mark on the bone, macroscopic observation is the main tool for recognising and identifying diseases.[36] We can say that, only after the technological availability of radiological examination[37]

and computerized axial tomography[38] – CAT scans – in the 1970s and 1980s, can we establish an autonomous discipline within Egyptology itself.

We can add today to these techniques; MRI (Magnetic Resonance Imaging), Imagiology (medical exploration through images like ecography, ultrasound probing) and DNA testing (short for deoxyribonucleic acid, the essence of genetic material in organisms).

From the 1970s onwards, bioegyptology has expanded as an autonomous field of research connecting archaeology, forensic anthropology, linguistics (reading rolls of linen around Egyptian bodies and engravings in amulets found with these bodies and any other inscription that is pertinent to the study of mummified bodies), medicine, botanic and many other sciences if we include specialized ones such as chemistry and geology.

The aim of this work is to synthesize information from ancient Egyptian daily life; everything that has been written upon it and analyzed until today, throughout the world, in different perspectives and several languages, thus giving a contribution for international research and also possible future contributions for medicine and Egyptology. The analysis of texts was done from the linguistic point of view and its interpretation has been reviewed already, in part, by some Egyptologists in the 20th century and even into the 21st century. Therefore we are driven here to gather the reading of some sections of medical prescriptions from these earlier translations, interpretations on them and also some notes, as well as the analysis of some hieroglyphic characters, (mainly the ones referring to important parts of the human body and some of the health concerns). We make a comparison of ancient Egyptian practices with present practices in medicine and pharmacy; analyzing the efficacy of medicinal properties scientifically proven on some Egyptian flora species (foreign and endemic) and their utilization in the prescribed treatments,[39] as well as the use of human ingredients, other animal and also mineral ones for the wellbeing of ancient Egyptians.

There are already some general publications on medicine in ancient Egypt that were used in the bibliography for this work; we are not trying to re-write the matter under the same perspective, or to take too long on linguistic matters either such as the specific hieroglyph for a specific body part or even fall under the same theories not yet certified such as the one on the *aaa* disease, '3',

[33] Ruffer, 1910.
[34] There is a prize from L'Académie Royale de Médecine de Belgique named Docteur Frans Jonckheere sur l'Histoire de la Médecine.
[35] Tilde Binger, from Copenhagen, a former preacher now professor of the Old Testament at the Department of Biblical Studies from Copenhagen University, http://www.ku.dk/aarbog/97/1/1220.html
[36] Notes taken from Prof. Eugénia Cunha in a session of Forensic Anthropology at the Instituto de Medicina Legal de Lisboa (Forensic Institute of Lisbon), February 2007. Prof. Eugénia Cunha is one of the authors of *Forensic Anthropology and Medicine: Complementary Sciences from Recovery to Cause of Death*, Humana Press, 2006.
[37] Wilhelm Conrad Röntgen (1845-1923) German physicist from Würzburg University, that in November 1895, produced and detected the electromagnetic radiation known as X-ray or Röntgen ray, which gave him the Nobel prize of Physics in 1901.

[38] Godfrey Newbold Hounsfield, from the UK, invented the first machine in 1967, and in 1968 the complete equipment, in 1972 he recorded the patent. In 1973 the famous Mayo Clinic, USA scans the brain and it is wanted by everyone. Hounsfield gets the Nobel Prize of Physiology and Medicine in 1979. The Nobel Committee describes Hounsfield as the central person in computerized axial tomography, a revolutionary radiological method, specifically in the research for nervous system diseases.
[39] Flora with magical properties studied by Wessely, 1931: 19-26.

We want to demonstrate that it is possible, in the near future, to complete the Egyptological analysis of the available sources of information, with new discoveries, to gain a perspective on the daily life in ancient Egypt of personal and public health concerns, in different specialties; some more important and known of the pharaonic civilization. To take an innovative approach and fluid approach; as the bioegyptology branch is still an embryo.

The progression of our knowledge of ancient Egyptian medicine has benefited from several elements of advancing technology, including new models and techniques of examining mummified remains, more precise translations of medical and magical papyri and a more detailed interpretation of some hieroglyphs. Seasonal archaeological expeditions help facilitate this knowledge. In the study of paleodisease, progression has been made in using non-invasive techniques. This is possible in some medical departments and Museums in the USA, Canada and Europe and in the National Research Centre of Cairo which works in collaborative projects with the KNH Centre of Manchester, UK.[40]

As Manuel Juaneda Magdalena states in his article *La Paleopatología en Egipto: pasado y presente:* " (...) Se han constituido corpos cientificos de primer orden (Manchester Museum Mummy Research Project, 1973) entre otros, para el estudio de las momias y que actualmente son un referencia con una meta muy clara: el abordaje científico e interdisciplinario de los restos momificados y establecer una metodología para cada investigación y fomentar el conocimiento de la enfermedad y de las condiciones de vida de las poblaciones en la antigüedad. (...)"[41]

The first woman to be professor of Egyptology in the UK and in charge of the Manchester Mummy Research for more than thirty years now (established in 1973), is Professor Rosalie David.[42]

She has done pioneering work in research using non-invasive techniques. Today, the KNH Centre for Biomedical Egyptology in Manchester is the world Centre for biomedical Egyptology. In the KNH, analysis are done on tissue samples, more than a thousand, hosted in the Mummy Tissue Bank,[43] with different provenances from around the world, allowing a more rapid development of biomedical Egyptology. Patterns of disease are studied, with special attention to schistosomiasis, with the future goal of developing detection techniques for immunological diseases, identifying more rapidly the causes and finding possible treatments as these diseases are still endemic to present Egypt.[44]

Even today, and according to Amal Samy Ibrahim, epidemiologist at the University of Cairo, this bacteria (schistosome) causes complications in gallbladder cancer which represents 30.8 % of all cancers in Egypt, 40 % in men, making it the most common cancer in this country, and Egypt has the highest rate of gall bladder cancer cases. This happens generally around 50 years of age. This disease makes it more difficult to treat this cancer as the patients attacked by this bacterium have some difficulty with chemotherapy treatments.[45]

In ancient Egypt they already recognised carcinomas (tumour, *aat*, ⌃◌, '*3t*) [46] but they were difficult to distinguish from other inflammations such as pustules, abscesses, blisters, pouches of fluid and cysts.[47]

There were both seasons of prosperity and famine as attested by some material found and some art depictions. In a cemetery from the reign of Ramesses II seventy skeletons were found and studied by the team of Manfred Bietak in the autumn of 2005[48] they were abnormally small and bad nutrition seems to have been the cause for this; adult women averaged only 1.40 m in height (from 1.37 to 1.45 m), and adult men were, on average, only 10 cm more (1.50 m). "Do written sources contradict archaeological findings?" A paradox, says Manfred Bietak: "Contemporary texts such as the *Anastasi II* and *Anastasi III* Papyri speak of the town splendor. There are even records where the king describes the prosperity of the population and he is praised". Written sources are therefore tendentious – as opposed to archaeological findings that are objective – "we must know how to interpret them", explains Bietak. The cooperation between Egyptology and scientific subjects becomes

---

[40] KNH Centre of Manchester http://www.knhcentre.manchester.ac.uk/ National Research Centre of Cairo
http://www.nrc.sci.eg/AboutUs/AboutUs.asp
[41] *Paleopathology in Egypt: past and present:* "(...) First class scientific Centers have been set up (Manchester Museum Mummy Research Project, 1973) among others, for the study of mummies that are presently a reference with a clear purpose: the scientific interdisciplinary approach to mummified remains and the establishment of a methodology for each investigation in promoting the knowledge of disease and daily life conditions of ancient populations", Magdalena, 2001.
[42] Some of her publications, among articles and books, both in paper and online are crucial for these studies for their scientific importance for all research in the paleopathology of ancient Egypt:
http://www.ancientegyptmagazine.com/mummy01.htm

[43] Lambert-Zazulak P., October 2003, The International Ancient Egyptian Mummy Tissue Bank at the Manchester Museum as a resource for the palaeoepidemiological study of schistosomiasis, World Archaeology, Volume 35, Number 2, pp. 223-240, Routledge
[44] The relation between prescriptions to treat these diseases and the plants used in them, even the unknown ones, as well as any evidence left in mummified bodies, are the object of research in an ongoing project of the KNH: Pharmacy in ancient Egypt,
http://www.knhcentre.manchester.ac.uk/research/pharmacyproject/
[45] Sheweita e O'Connor, 1999.
[46] Nunn, 1996: 217.
[47] This differentiation is possible after specific readings that led to the work presented at the Pharmacy and Medicine in ancient Egypt Conference at Manchester on September 2008,
http://www.knhcentre.manchester.ac.uk/newsandevents/pharmacyconfer ence/index.asp, about the paragraphs 857 - 877 from the Ebers Papyrus following, among others the work of Baillard, 1998: 9-61.
[48] http://www.auaris.at/html/index_en.html,
http://homepage.univie.ac.at/
elisabeth.trinkl/forum/forum0999/12tell.htm

more important, determines Bietak. Archaeology can point out social structures outside society says Bietak.

The inscription on the "Famine Stela" in Aswan, at the island of Sehel, engraved by the priests of Khnum at Elephantine, states that, king Djoser, at the suggestion of his counselor Imhotep, called all Egyptians to cultivate the land belonging to the Khnum temple in order to end the famine in Egypt. The text was written part under Ptolemy V Epiphanes: more than two thousand years after the death of king Djoser, and says:[49]

"I was in mourning on my throne,
Those of the palace were in grief,
My heart was in great affliction,
Because Hapy had failed to come in time
In a period of seven years.
Grain was scant,
Kernels were dried up,
Scarce was every kind of food.
Every man robbed his twin,
Those who entered did not go.
Children cried,
Youngsters fell,
The hearts of the old were grieving;
Legs drawn up, they hugged the ground,
Their arms clasped about them.
Courtiers were needy,
Temples were shut,
Shrines covered with dust,
Everyone was in distress."[50]

Between 51 and 49 BC, Egypt suffered a famine period due to bad crops caused by the drought. Ptolemy XIII signed a decree on October 27th, 50 BC which forbade all shipments of cereals to the exterior with the exception of Alexandria. In 1889, Charles Wilbour discovered an inscription on the island of Sehel, which recorded this famine as lasting for seven years under the reign of Djoser.

Daily life was therefore a preparation for the afterlife (a much better life, an ancient Egyptian belief based on their own writing); with gods to whom oracles were dedicated, requests were made and spells were prepared with, considering that, in the Greco-Roman Period the average life expectancy was of 25 years, for the ones surviving birth, between 35 and 40 years of age for those passing the first year of life, and close to 45 for those able to reach 5 years of age.[51]

This demonstrates the difficulties of survival for the majority of ancient Egyptian people, compounded by deficient hygiene standards, plagues grassing in the country, harsh and aggressive climate conditions; the heat

and the desert winds. In addition, areas of still water of the Nile and its channels were sources of procreation for pathological microorganisms.

3. Specific existing bibliography – some important examples

At present there are Egyptologists, paleopathologists, doctors and scientists from different countries and nationalities and different academic backgrounds that have specialized and become interested in ancient Egyptian medicine and are writing about it.[52] Some works are referenced below as examples among many bibliographic references used, showing the specificity of some authors in their research. Those referenced below being more general about health, medicine and prescriptions of prophylactic-palliative characteristics (used ingredients, magic as an element and all the notions given to us by ancient Egyptians). A summary is made here after the headings, focusing on some notes taken and on most important aspects in our opinion:

Ebeid, N. I. *Egyptian Medicine in the Days of the Pharaohs*, The General Egyptian Book Organization, Cairo, 1999

In this work from the doctor Nabil Ebeid about medical practices in the pharaonic era, the author describes some of the analysis done on mummies in pages 28 to 55; talks about priests, anatomy, Sekhmet and surgery in pages 70 to 137, with special focus on tumours in pages 102 to 116. The following sections are about orthopaedics, women's diseases and internal medicine, where we find information about the liver. He goes on with references to teeth diseases and their therapeutics, diet, cosmetics and medicine at the workplace. After that we have chapters on hygiene and sanitation in ancient Egypt, and reference to health and medicine related gods and also on physical deformities. He finishes this work with a chapter on mummification and its importance for medical science and Egyptian historiography mentioning the main collaborators on this. The bibliography indicated by this author, (1999), allows any ancient Egyptian medicine researcher valid information on complementary sources of information.

Nunn, John, F. *Ancient Egyptian Medicine*, British Museum, London, University of Oklahoma Press, Norman, Oklahoma, 1996

In this work by the doctor John Nunn, recently retired from supervision of the Anaesthetic Department of the Medical Research Council in London, a member of the EES,[53] translator of some Egyptian medical papyri, and for twenty years dedicated to the study of medicine in ancient Egypt. There are excellent visual diagrams

---

[49] Lichtheim, 1997: 130-134.
[50] Lichtheim, 1980: 94-100.
[51] Tunny, 2001: 120,
http://www.utexas.edu/depts/classics/documents/Life.html, Bagnall 2006, 90, 104; Nerlich, 2001.

[52] Special Note: All German referenced Works here are only quoted because of their importance for this study but those were not browsed.
[53] Egypt Exploration Society founded in 1882, presently at 3, Doughty Mews, London.

presented about body parts' names in hieroglyphic in pages 46, 47 and 217 to 226. The author talks about Egyptian medical papyri, going through human physiology and the diseases affecting ancient Egyptians, from which we can gather much information.

Further in this work he goes through the role of magic in medicine, showing charts of the medical-magical 'job' as shown in pages 118, 119, 121 and 210 to 216. Also presented here is a relationship between mineral, animal and vegetable pharmacopoeia, with associated charts on pages 136 to 162. Finally a list of traumatic diseases and medical specialties is presented. The bibliography mentioned is also interesting, because, besides Egyptological work, he mentions work done by doctors with knowledge of Egyptology.

Manniche, Lise, *An Ancient Egyptian Herbal*, British Museum Publications, London, 1989.

As medical papyri are one of the main sources of information for our work because of the medical prescriptions described in them, it is essential to mention this work, as Lise Manniche includes in it a chapter on the ancient Egyptian flora used in medical prescriptions. Vegetables are one of the groups of ingredients used in the preparation of prescriptions both curative and preventive, it is therefore crucial to try and cross plants' names and descriptions in the medical papyri and in other sources of information and their use in medical care.[54]

Illustrated in black and white drawings, this work starts to mention the use of medicinal plants in page 58. A complete herbarium lists plant information with its Latin name, its ancient Egyptian and Coptic names[55] and also in Greek and contemporary Arabic, when possible. This is enough to investigate these plants in the present times; to determine their characteristics and active substances which are now reproduced in pharmaceutical laboratories by chemical methods. Thus some can be identified and of course, there are many that we cannot identify as well. Dioscorides work is also cross referenced to give us more information and opportunities for comparisons.

Bardinet, Thierry, *Les papyrus médicaux de l'Égypte pharaonique: Traduction intégrale et commentaire*, Penser la Médecine, Librairie Arthème Fayard, Paris, 1995

In this excellent work, continuing the work done by Gustave Lefebvre,[56] and completing some issues that Lefebvre did not mention, Bardinet starts with the role of the priests/doctors fighting diseases, using magic. He continues with hieroglyphic definitions of name concepts, talks about pathogenic elements, anatomy theories and the largest part of his work is the study of the medical texts. In these texts we can analyze, in detail, from the French, some expressions and content of the medical prescriptions. The knowledge of the medical papyri and their different translations paying attention to the original ones where the hieroglyphic can be compared is of extreme importance, but the contemporary cross-examining of these oldest translations with new insights from medical science brings together more accurate conclusions.

Ruffer, Marc Armand, *Studies in the Paleopathology of Egypt*, ed. Roy L. Moodie, The University of Chicago Press, Chicago, 1921

Sir Marc Armand Ruffer (1859-1917) was the Pioneer of paleopathology[57] and, although this publication dates from 1921 gathering work done by Ruffer since 1909[58] until shortly before his death, it is still a crucial work for those studying the patterns of health in ancient Egyptians. In it we find records of examinations that Ruffer did to several Egyptian mummies over the years, with particular remarks, as they reflect precise conclusions; they are real 'autopsies' giving us an insight of what afflicted ancient Egyptians. He analyzed all kinds of human tissue; skin, muscle, nerves, organs, bones from both whole bodies and disarticulated body parts from mummified Egyptian material. He was a Professor of Bacteriology in the Cairo Medical School, and he defined paleopathology as "the science of disease that can be demonstrated in ancient human and animal tissue remains."

The histology of ancient Egyptian tissue material was described for the first time by Ruffer in 1911, as he found *Schistosoma haematobium* eggs in a mummy from the XXth Dynasty. Until the 1990's, the analysis methods included radiology, CAT scans, endoscopy, macroscopic observation, electron microscopy and serology. Several infections were diagnosed: schistosomiasis, dracontiasis

---

[54] The Pharmacy of ancient Egypt Project from the KNH Centre in Manchester is pursuing this cross-referenced work to try to determine which are the 'unknown' plants referred to in medical papyri and their efficacy in medical prescriptions.

[55] Coptic has its origin in the expression *het-ka-ptah* which means palace of the *ka* from Ptah
(http://www.coptic.net/lessons/CopticSlideShow.txt), name of the temple in Memphis that was spread all over Egypt. The Greeks changed it to *aigyptos*; Egypt for us in the Western world, as its actual name in Arabic today is Misr.

[56] Lefebvre, G, *Essai sur la médecine égyptienne de l'époque pharaonique*, Paris, 1956.
[57] The term was established in 1892 by an American doctor, R. W. Shufeldt, from two Greek words: *palaios*, ancient, and *pathos*, pain/suffering.
[58] This publication contains several articles by the author: Ruffer, M., A., *Remarks on the histology and pathological anatomy of Egyptian mummies*, Cairo Scientific Journal, 1910; 4: 3-7; *Note on the Presence of 'Bilharzia Haematobia' in Egyptian Mummies of the XXth Dynasty 1250-1000 BC*. BMJ 1: 16; *On arterial lesions found in Egyptian mummies*, Journal Pathology Bacteriology 1911; 15: 453-462; *Note on an eruption resembling that of variola in the skin of a mummy of the twentieth dynasty (1200-1100 B.C.)*; *Histological Studies on Egyptian Mummies (Mémoires présentés a l'institut Egyptien)*, Le Caire, 6, Fasc. 3 (Mars, 1911); Marc Armand Ruffer, Arnoldo Rietti, *On osseous lesions in ancient Egyptians*, The Journal of Pathology and Bacteriology, 1911; *Pathological note on the royal mummies of the Cairo Museum*.

(Guinea worm), tricocefaliasis, ascaridaysis and bone tuberculosis as prevalent diseases in ancient Egyptians. The recent introduction of molecular identification methods (PCR) brings new light to the study of paleopathology.

David, Rosalie and Archbold, Rick, *Conversations with Mummies, New Light on the Ancient Egyptians*, Harper Collins, London, 2000

In this work Rosalie David and Rick Archbold give us a perspective on the path undergone by biomedicine in Egyptology, particularly regarding the Manchester Mummy Project but also illustrating other cases of mummies' analysis important to this research. The 1975 examination, broadcasted by BBC, was decisive for this branch of Egyptology in the scientific society and in the international community of Egyptologists. This is a complete manual of autopsies of mummified bodies which leads us through the whole process, bearing all the details in mind, from the body itself to its bandages, footwear, jewellery, and even prosthetics. Several questions are presented referring to the autopsy made and achieved results. Obvious references to examinations on mummies done in the early 1900's are included (1908), also in Manchester, by Margaret Murray, including the case of The Two Brothers, Khnumnakht e Nekhtankh, which was carried out by the present Manchester Mummy Project.[59] This work continues with Napoleon's first Egypt trip and mentions others such as Denon, remembering the 'dinner parties' by Pettigrew, other mummy autopsies, the work of Sir Flinders Petrie and Elliot Smith and the discovery of Tutankhamun's by Carter.

The mummification procedures are described as well, with references to the instruments, ceramic vases and other 'accessories' such as the shouabtis.[60] Sarcophagi and masks, bandages and portraits of Roman Egypt in the sarcophagi, all these were part of the complex system of identity preservation for the afterlife. A recent attempt to mummify a body in order to get to some conclusions is also mentioned.

The work of Cockburn is mentioned, as he has undertaken important examinations on mummified tissues, Nakht in particular. The autopsy done in Paris in 1976 to the mummy of Ramesses II is also mentioned.

The information about the 1881 discovery of a mass grave in Thebes containing several royal mummies is given as an important piece of information for the history of this field, the Valley of the Kings and its importance is also discussed.

A reference to the mummy of DjedMaatiuesankh from the Royal Ontario Museum in Canada is made, including examinations undertaken on the mummy, applied techniques, radiography and CAT scan, all the surrounding objects and a possible lifetime path is given.

Following this we have a description of the DNA techniques which were even able to identify parasitical presence in viscera remains. The investigation going on at Manchester allows for the study of malaria among other infectious diseases.

Showing important images, this work refers summarily but in a very professional and explanatory way, the process of mummification from the remains we have in the present allied to the present available techniques.

Pinch, Geraldine, *Magic in Ancient Egypt*, University of Texas Press, Austin, 1994

This is an essential work in the study of magic in ancient Egypt and it starts with looking at the concept of magic and its meaning to the ancient Egyptians, in mythology and the essence of the word *heka*. It continues establishing the connection between the myth and magic, similarities and differences; demons and spirits; priests' practices; written magic and the power of the word; magical techniques; wax figures and others used in magical *performance*; the amulets, essential to life, health and after death. It describes also the medical-magical conceptions connected to fecundity; establishes the parallel between medicine and magic; continues with funerary myths, practices and concepts of life after death and ends with the contribution of magic in ancient Egypt to civilizations after them.
It was very important to the elaboration of this work and it served as a basis for further research through its bibliography and notes.

---

[59]http://www.ancientegypt.co.uk/manchester/pages/the%20two%20brot hers.htm, R. David (2007) The Two Brothers Death and the afterlife in Ancient Egypt. *Rutherford Press, Liverpool*
[60]They did all the work in the afterlife for the deceased; hard work like agriculture. Referenced in Pinch, 1994: 158.

Chapter 1
Sources of Information; Medical and Magical Papyri

As sources of information for the study of medical-magical practices in ancient Egypt we have included (even those that are not quoted but that were used to draw conclusions and understand better the ancient Egyptian society):
-Egyptian Papyri in different writings, (hieroglyphic, demotic, hieratic, Coptic, including Greek), ostraca, general literature (personal letters), all of which include medical or magical content.[61]
-Mummified and skeletal human remains.
-Painted and sculptured artistic depictions, in tombs, objects found in excavations that show physical deformities, traumas or diseases.
-Foreign travellers' diaries that, although they are subsequent to the pharaonic era, show characteristics and habits that are persistent in Egypt today, since ancient times.
-General literature showing evidence of diseases (again, personal letters),[62] food habits, periods of famine and abundance caused by war or natural events such as the annual flood.

Medical and magical Papyri

Medical and magical Papyri related to health, and also mummification	Date found	Place of discvery
Berlin 3027		
Berlin 3038	c. 1827	Saqqara
Edwin Smith	c. 1860	Thebes
Ebers	c. 1862	Thebes
Kahun UC 32057 (gynaecological)	c. 1889	Lahun
Ramesseum III, IV e V e VIII a XVI	c. 1896	behind the Ramesseum at Thebes
Hearst	c. 1899	Deir el-Ballas, south Dendera
London Papyrus 10059[63]	?	Thebes
Papyri Chester Beatty	c. 1928	Deir el-Medina
Carlsberg VIII	c. 1939	?
Brooklyn 47218-02, 47218-138 e 47218-48 e 47218-48-85	?	?
Insinger	?	?
Berlin 3033 – Westcar	c. 1825	?
IFAO Deir el-Medina 1	1928	Deir el-Medina
Leiden I 343-I 345	beginning 19th century	Thebes
Schøyen MS 2634/3	1969	Alexandria ?
Tebtunis	1900	Fayoum
Yale CtYBR 2081	1966	?
Papyrus Louvre[64]	1953	?
Rubensohn (Berlin 10456)[65]	1908	Abusir or Elefantine
Vindob 3873	1821	Alexandria
Turin 54003[66]		
Yearnymous Londinensis	?	?
Louvre E 4864[67]	?	?
Borgia	1778	Fayoum

---

[61] Lists with information on medical-magical papyri used: University College London: http://www.digitalegypt.ucl.ac.uk/med/healingpapyri.html; http://www.medizinische-papyri.de/html/medizinische_papyri.html; The Papyrus Carlsberg Collection, Copenhagen: http://www.hum.ku.dk/cni/papcoll/index.html; Center for the Tebtunis Papyri, University of California, Bancroft Library, Berkeley, California: http://tebtunis.berkeley.edu/collection/index.html; Yale University Beinecke Rare Book and Manuscript Library: http://www.library.yale.edu/beinecke/brblsear/aboutpap.htm#LDO; The Schøyen Collection: http://schoyencollection.com/smallercollect.htm#2634; University of Charleston: http://www.cofc.edu/~piccione/medbase.html; as listed in the bibliography.

[62] Pinch, 1994: 150.

[63] http://www.britishMuseumm.org/research/search_the_collection_database/search_object_details.aspx

[64] Irá ser estudado e as suas conclusões publicadas após a exposição entre 6 de Junho e 6 de Agosto de 2007 no Museum do Louvre, segundo o seu curador, Marc Étienne.

[65] Published in Rubensohn, O., Elephantine Papyri; Ägyptische Urkunden aus den königlichen Museen zu Berlin: Griechische Urkunden, Sonderheft, Berlin, 1907.

[66] Borghouts, 1978: 23; http://digilander.libero.it/Egitto_Antico/SDP_CompendioPapiri3.pdf.

[67] Musée du Louvre: http://cartelfr.louvre.fr/cartelfr/visite?srv=car_not_frame&idNotice=3360

Medical and magical Papyri related to health, and also mummification	Date found	Place of discvery
Bulaq 3 Mummification	?	?
Louvre 5158 Mummification	?	?
Carlsberg 13 e 14 (dream interpretation) *Carlsberg* 67 (prayer to request a cure from Sobek, at the Fayoum)	?	?
Chassinat Coptic IFAO[68]		

---

[68] Chassinat, 1921.

1.1. *Papyrus de Kahun* UC 32057

The *Kahun Papyrus* was discovered by Sir William Matthew Flinders Petrie in April 1889 near Lahun,[69] near the Fayoum oasis. Flinders Petrie was the founder of the British School of Archaeology in Egypt and first Edwards Professor of Egyptology in the University College of London;[70] he was awarded Knightship in 1923. Today, there is a Museum with his name[71] where we can see, among many priceless artifacts, human samples of tissue such as hair, instruments that may have been used in surgery, objects of cosmetics and unguent jars.

Flinders Petrie published *Kahun, Gurob and Hawara*,[72] with a description of the excavation site, drawings of the objects found, as well as plants and some notes about the flora and daily life.

The so-called gynecological Papyrus (Kahun) is today at the University College of London in a poor state of preservation. Dated from the XIIth Dynasty (c. 1850-1700 BC), the reign of Amenemhat III, it is very fragmentated. It was published with a *facsimile* and translated to English by Griffith in 1898 and then by Stevens in 1975; it deals essentially with gynecological issues. It will not be the subject of detailed study in this work.[73]

1.2. *Papyrus Edwin Smith*

James Henry Breasted, born in 1822,[74] was director of the Oriental Institute of Chicago, and he published this papyrus translation into English in 1930 with a *facsimile*, transcription, comments and introduction. This volume was put together with some medical notes prepared by Arno B. Luckhardt. Until today, Breasted's edition is still the only publication considered as a complete work on this text.

The papyrus belongs to the New York Academy of Medicine and was exhibited in the Metropolitan Museum of Art of New York in an exhibition about The Art of Medicine in Ancient Egypt (2005-2006).[75] Dated from the New Kingdom (c. 1550 BC) and found in a Theban tomb, it was put up for sale around 1860 by Mustafa Agha and, in 1862, was bought by Edwin Smith, an American resident in Egypt. When he died in 1906, his daughter donated the Papyrus to the New York Historical Society. It mentions diseases and surgery cases, 62 in total, fourteen with known treatments, and 48 without mentioning any treatment, maybe chronic diseases difficult to treat or even unknown diseases. It has seventeen pages and it was found in the tomb of a doctor.[76] It deals with the examinations of patients undertaken by the doctor and the majority of the examples given are of trauma cases. The word "brain" is used for the first time to mention the organ in question: " (…) Smashing his skull, and rending open the brain of his skull," it means the smash is large, opening to the interior of his skull, to the membrane enveloping his brain, so that it breaks open his fluid in the interior of his head."[77]

1.3. *Papyrus Ebers*

Magic is effective together with medicine. Medicine is effective together with magic, according to the texts

---

[69] Between Beni Suef and the Fayoum, el-Lahun village was in the Nile west bank close to the Fayoum. Hundreds of texts written in hieratic were found here, in the ancient village of Ro-henet, which means "mouth of the channel" and is translated to Coptic as Illahun.

[70] Chair after Amelia Edwards, deceased in 1892; in January 1893, William Matthew Flinders Petrie, her favourite archaeologist in Egypt, became the first Edwards Professor of Egyptian Archaeology and Philology, at 39 years of age. This Chair was offered to the University College London, with preference over Oxford and Cambridge, because, at that time, the UCL was the only place in the UK offering a Chair to women: http://www.digitalegypt.ucl.ac.uk/archaeology/edwards.html

[71] http://www.petrie.ucl.ac.uk/

[72] Flinders Petrie, W. M., London, 1890

[73] Women's diseases, childbirth and STD were the objects of an article written for the Second International Conference for Young Egyptologists at Lisbon, October 2006; a CD version of the Proceedings will be published soon (*To prevent, treat and cure love in ancient Egypt*).

[74] A curious coincidence: the 'official' birth of Egyptology.

[75] http://www.metMuseumm.org/special/Art_Medicine_Egypt/medicine_more.asp

[76] David, 2008: 188; Sanchez, 2007.

[77] Feldman, 1999; Bardinet, 1995: 236-237, 497.

prescribing treatments; these texts protect the doctor practicing the treatment.[79] At the same time as Papyrus Edwin Smith another Papyrus was bought in 1872 by Egyptologist George Ebers who gave it his name. In 1875, Ebers published a *facsimile*, but it was the Norwegian Bendix Ebbell in 1937 who concluded the most exhaustive study of this Papyrus to date.[80] It contains 877 medical treatments covering physical, mental and spiritual diseases. The *Ebers Papyrus* has references to eye diseases, gastrointestinal, head, skin, and specific still unidentified diseases; *aaa*, probably *ancylostomiasis* (hookworm - endemic to ancient Egypt).[81]

This Papyrus has 110 pages and dates to 1534 BC, the reign of Amenhotep I.[82] It contains spells, a section on gastric diseases, intestinal parasites, skin, anus diseases, a small treatise on the heart, and some prescriptions thought to have been used by gods. It continues with migraine treatments, urinary tract disturbances, coughs, hair conditions, burns and different wounds, extremities (fingers and toes), tongue, teeth, ears nose and throat, gynaecological conditions and a last section on what is thought to be tumours.

Paragraphs 1-3 have a series of magical spells to protect the patient from surgical intervention in the diagnosis and treatment. Following we find a large section on gastric diseases and parasitic and intestinal infestations are described in paragraphs 50-85.[83] Skin diseases have three categories: irritative, exfoliative and ulcerative, in paragraphs 90-95 and 104-118.

Diseases of the anus are covered in paragraphs 132-164[84] until paragraph 187. Some diseases are more difficult to translate. They may have recognizable symptoms such as an obstruction, but they can use a specific word such as *wekhedw* or *aaa*. Paragraphs 242-247 have the description of some prescriptions thought to have been used by gods.[85] Paragraph 250 is all about migraines. In paragraph 251 a drug is mentioned: "knowledge of what is done with *degem* (probably *ricinus* oil), as something found in ancient texts and useful to man."[86] Paragraphs 261-283 deal with the urine flux and medicines to "make the heart receive bread"[87] Paragraphs 305-335 have medicines for coughing and diseases of the knee. The rest is about hair (437-476), liver diseases (477-481), trauma wounds, burns, flesh wounds (482-529) and treatment of extremities.

Paragraphs 627-696 deal with the relaxing and straightening of the *metu* channels. The meaning of *metu* is dubious; they can be blood vessels, tendons or any other channel of fluid or ligament in the body. The Papyrus continues with tongue diseases (697-704), skin conditions (708-721), teeth (739-750), ear, nose and throat (761-781) and gynaecological issues (783-839). It is somewhat similar to *The Edwin Smith Papyrus* in the treatment of limbs hardened and painful, and also similar to *Kahun Papyrus* in the gynaecological issues.

1.4. *Papyrus Hearst*

Housed at the Bancroft Library, University of California, it was discovered at Deir el-Ballas in Upper Egypt, south of Dendera, in 1899, and it became a property of the California American Expedition (Hearst Egyptian Expedition) when George Andrew Reisner brought it in 1901. Dated from the New Kingdom (c. 1500 BC), it was published by George Andrew Kingsner (1867-1942), in Leipzig in 1905, then by W. Wreszinski, *Der Londoner medizinische Papyrus (und der Papyrus Hearst)*, Leipzig, 1912, in: Medizin der alten Ägypter, II, Leipzig 1912; e em Deines, H. von, Grapow, H. and Westendorf, W., *Grundriss der Medizin der alten Ägypter*, Berlin, Akademie-Verlag, 1954-63, 1973. It has 260 medical formulae, and deals with general clinical cases. Some of the texts (96) are found in *The Ebers Papyrus*.

It has eighteen pages, concentrating on urinary tract treatments, blood, hair and snake and scorpion bites. Written in hieratic, its prescriptions go from "a tooth that has fallen out" (column I, l. 7) to "medicine to treat the lung" (column IV, l. 8) and even human bites (column Ll de II. 6-7) and also bites from pigs and hippopotamus (column Ll de XVI. 5-7). This Papyrus is in very good condition. It has also a chapter on orthopaedics.

Fragment 8 deals specifically with *metu* diseases.[88]

1.5. *London Papyrus* BM 10059

Housed at the British Museum since the beginning of the 20th century,[89] it belonged first to the Royal Institute of London. Dated from the XIXth Dynasty (c.1300 BC) and published by W. Wreszinski[90] it has some magical formulae, with spiritual and magical texts (demon cast-away spells);[91] spells against swellings, some unidentified diseases, one for the placenta, dermatological diseases, eye diseases, against haemorrhages (in pregnant women) and burns. It has some 62 prescriptions from which only 25 are medical.[92]

---

[79] Bardinet, 1995: 39-59

[80] Nunn, 1996: 30. Ebers, G. M., Stern, L., *Papyrus Ebers*, Facsimile with a partial translation, 2 volumes, 1875; Joachim, H., Reimer, Berlin, G., *Papyros Ebers*, The first complete translation from the Egyptian, 1890; B. Ebbell, *The papyrus Ebers, The greatest Egyptian Medical document*, Copenhagen, Levin & Munksgaard, 1937.

[81] Davis, 2000; Kloos, 2002.

[82] Nunn, 1996: 31.

[83] Bryan, 1974: 50.

[84] Nunn, 1996: 32.

[85] Nunn, 1996: 33. Bryan, 1974: 45.

[86] Nunn, 1996: 33.

[87] Nunn, 1996: 33.

[88] Egypt's Golden Age, 1982: 295.

[89] http://www.thebritishMuseumm.ac.uk/explore/highlights/highlight_objects/aes/t/the_london_medical_papyrus.aspx

[90] W. Wreszinski, *Der Londoner medizinische Papyrus (und der Papyrus Hearst)*: Medizin der alten Ägypter, Band II, Leipzig 1912; e em Deines, H. von, Grapow, H. e Westendorf, W., *Grundriss der Medizin der alten Ägypter*, Berlin, Akademie-Verlag, 1954-63, 1973.

[91] Borghouts, 1978: 21, 23.

[92] Leitz, 1999: 51-52.

We can also find a spell to cast away flies in the Nile banks when building or planting there. There is, in this Papyrus, evidence of interchanging with foreign cultures,[93] in particular there is mention of new vegetable and mineral ingredients being increasingly used in New Kingdom Egypt.[94]

1.6. *Berlin Papyrus* 3038

Housed in the Berlin Museum since 1827, it is probably dated to the reign of Ramesses II, from the XIXth Dynasty and it was discovered in the beginning of the 19th century in a Saqqara tomb. It was then sold to William IV from Prussia with other items in 1827 and then went to the Berlin Museum. Wreszinski made a translation to German in 1909. It has 24 pages (21 in the recto and 3 in the verso).[95]

It deals with general clinical cases and it is similar to *Papyrus Ebers*. It contains 25 pages and 240 prescriptions, three of the pages are written in a different language. A large part of its index consists of a reproduction, word by word, with many mistakes and careless copy of some paragraphs from the *Ebers Papyrus* and also *Hearst Papyrus*. This includes sections on rheumatisms, a treatise on the heart, similar to the one on the *Ebers Papyrus*, and a note about its origin, more detailed than the one found in the *Ebers Papyrus*.

1.7. *Chester Beatty Papyri*

These are a collection of fragments discovered in 1928 in the working village of Deir el-Medina (Western Thebes) and are preserved in different places: Institut Français d'Archéologie Orientale (IFAO), Cairo; Ashmolean Museum, Oxford; Chester Beatty Library and Gallery, Dublin and the British Museum. The London fragments were donated by the industrial millionaire Sir Alfred Chester Beatty and are in a bad state of preservation, although some restoration work was done on them.[96] They were initially published by Gardiner[97] and Jonckheere,[98] and are part of the *Grundriss* (German).[99]

They are dated from the XIXth Dynasty, and they belonged to a family of scribes at Deir el-Medina. They include prescriptions to treat diseases of the anus, spells against migraines and some prescriptions and spells still unknown.

Chester Beatty V (BM 10685), in its third section, has some magical formulae against migraines; *Chester Beatty* VI (BM 10686), consisting of eight pages, divided into 41 paragraphs, is almost entirely dedicated to anus diseases and also has some spells for unknown diseases; *Chester Beatty* VII (BM 10687), has magical formulae against scorpion bites; *Chester Beatty* VIII, (BM 10688), the less interesting one, has a prescription for an unknown disease, among magical texts; *Chester Beatty* XI has spells for good health, including the Tale of Isis and Ra (BM 10691). There are others which also have spells for good health; *Chester Beatty* XII, (BM 10692), *Chester Beatty* XIII, (BM 10693), *Chester Beatty* XIV, (BM 10694), *Chester Beatty* XV, (BM 10695), from which only one page is preserved with some lines on prescriptions to destroy the "mouth thirst"; *Chester Beatty* XVI, (BM 10696) and *Chester Beatty* XVIII, (BM 10698).[100]

1.8. *Carlsberg Papyrus* VIII

These fragments, written in Hieratic, are housed at the Carsten Niebuhr Institute of Copenhagen. They are dated probably from between the XIXth and the XXth Dynasties, but it is reported to the XIIth Dynasty.[101]

It was first published by Iversen,[102] then by Buchheim,[103] and later on by Grapow.[104]

It has some notes in the verso about the Egyptian origin of birth prognosis, it deals with obstetrics and is similar to both the *Kahun Papyrus* and the *Berlin Papyrus*.[105] It also refers to some pregnancy problems, the determination of the fetus' sex and the probability of conception. In the Papyrus' recto there is a medical treatise dealing with eye diseases, it is in a bad state of preservation and almost a copy, page for page from the same section on the Ebers Papyrus.[106]

1.9. *Brooklyn Papyri* 47218-02, 47218-138 e 47218-48 e 47218-85

The place where these papyri were discovered is still unknown. There was a translation into French undertaken by Serge Sauneron which was published after his death, in 1989. These are housed at the Brooklyn Museum of New York.

These papyri are dated to the end of the XXXth Dynasty or beginning of the Ptolemaic Period but are written in

[93] Leitz, 1999: 61.
[94] Ritner, 2000: 107-117
[95] First studied by Passalacqua, then by H. Brugsch in 1855, Lepsius in 1865, and Wreszinski, W. *Der grosse medizinische Papyrus des Berliner Museums (Papyrus Berlin 3038)*. Leipzig: J. C. Hinrichs, 1909, Jonckheere in 1958, Ghalioungui in 1983 and Leca in 1988.
[96] Nunn, 1996: 36.
[97] Gardiner, A.H., *Hieratic Papyri in the British Museum, Third Series*, Chester Beatty Papyrus, British Museum, London, 1935.
[98] Jonckheere, F. *Le papyrus médical Chester Beatty*, La Médecine Égyptienne, 2, Fondation Égyptologique Reine Elisabeth, Brussels, 1947.
[99] Grapow (dir.), *Grundriss der Medizin der Alter Ägypter*, Berlin, 1954-1963 (com suplementos, 1973).

[100] Nunn, 1996: 37.
[101] Iversen, 1939: 4; Nunn, 1996: 39.
[102] Iversen, 1939.
[103] Buchheim, Liselotte, *Das Buch von den Augen und die Geburtsprognosen. Zwanzig Jahre Papyrus Carlsberg VIII*, Die medizinische Welt 15: 787-8, 1960.
[104] Grapow (dir.), *Grundriss der Medizin der Alter Ägypter*, Berlin, 1954-1963 (com suplementos, 1973).
[105] Iversen, 1939: 5.
[106] Iversen, 1939: 4; Nunn, 1996: 39.

Middle Kingdom style. They are about snake bites and treatment formulae to expel the venom from the body.[107]

1.10. Other Papyri

Ramesseum Papyri III, IV, V and VIII to XVI

Ramesseum Papyri III (BM 10756), IV (BM 10757) e V (BM 10758) e VIII (BM 10761) a XVI; (BM 10762, BM 10763, BM 10764, BM 10765, BM 10766, BM 10767, BM 10768, BM 10769) are housed at the British Museum. These were discovered by Quibell in 1896 in a wooden box at the bottom of a shaft, under some bricks, behind the Ramesseum at Thebes.[108] Some of which were studied and published by Gardiner in 1955, then by Barns in 1956 and also by the *Grundriss*.[109]

They contain sections about eye diseases, gynaecology, muscles and nerves, para-obstetrics practices and also paediatrics. Gardiner states that they may date from the XIIIth Dynasty, to the beginning of the Second Intermediate Period, written probably around 1900 BC, and dated from the same time as *Kahun Papyrus*.[110]

Ramesseum Papyri III and IV are magical-medical texts for mother and child.[111] *Ramesseum Papyrus* IV is very similar to *Kahun Papyrus*; it has many prescriptions about giving birth, how to protect the newborn at the day of his or her birth, the viability of the infant (life expectancy), and a contraceptive formula using crocodile dung. This ends similarly to the one on the *Kahun Papyrus*.[112]

Ramesseum Papyrus V has some prescriptions on the *metu*, being in a bad state of preservation as the beginning and end of the Papyrus are missing, but it has about twenty prescriptions on how to treat hardened limbs.[113] This Papyrus is written in cursive hieroglyphic, not Hieratic.[114] *Ramesseum Papyrus* VIII has a text on migraines.

Ramesseum Papyrus IX has some rituals on how to protect a house from magic, spirits and snakes. *Ramesseum Papyrus* X has magical spells on how to protect your limbs from snake bites. *Ramesseum Papyrus* XI has love spells and *Ramesseum Papyrus* XII has invocations to demons to treat fevers. *Ramesseum Papyri* XIII and XIV have some healing texts not yet studied. *Ramesseum Papyrus* XV has some spells to protect the body and *Papyrus* XVI has more spells against snakes and bad dreams.

Insinger Papyrus

The *Insinger Papyrus* is published in several works[115] and is dated from the Ptolemaic Period (304-30 BC). It mentions problems that arise from an unhealthy diet and a non-advisable lifestyle, stating what are the long term effects of the abuse of alcohol in ancient Egypt, the hangover of the morning after is mentioned using the French name hairache (*mal aux cheveux*); speaks also about obesity, that was not controlled or criticized:

" *The life that controls excess is a life according to a wise man's heart.*
Vegetables and natron are the best foods that can be found.
Illness befalls a man because the food harms him.
He who eats too much bread will suffer illness.
He who drinks too much wine lies down in a stupor.
All kinds of ailments are in the limbs because of overeating.
He who is moderate in his manner of life, his flesh is not disturbed.
Illness does not burn him who is moderate in food.
Poverty does not take hold of him who controls himself in purchasing.
His belly does not relieve itself in the street because of the food in it. "[116]
It also states that amulets and spells will only work by the hidden power of the god that acts upon the world.[117] This may refer to the practitioner/magician.

Berlin Papyrus 3033 – Westcar Papyrus

Papyrus containing a series of magical tales, probably recorded in the Old Kingdom, being dated from the Hyksos Period in ancient Egypt, where a magician shows his skills in the king's court.[118] In the tale called *The Birth of the Royal Children,* the text shows us how a delivery was performed.[119] Published by A. M. Blackman,[120] a transcription from the *Papyrus* includes comments on the hieroglyphic and state of preservation of the Papyrus with images from the original that will probably be the most ancient record of a magical practice, c. 2000 BC

Papyrus IFAO Deir el-Medina 1

At the workmen's village of *Deir el-Medina* many texts were found in Papyrus and ostraca. Some are housed presently at the Institut Français d'Archaéologie Orientale (IFAO), in Cairo, others are at the Ashmolean Museum in Oxford, Chester Beatty Library and Gallery in Dublin and at the British Museum in London.

---

[107] Nunn, 1996: 40.
[108] Nunn, 1996: 39.
[109] Barns, J. W. B., *Five Ramesseum Papyri*, The Griffith Institute, Oxford, 1956; Grapow (dir.), *Grundriss der Medizin der Alter Ägypter*, Berlin, 1954-1963 (with supplements, 1973).
[110] Nunn, 1996: 39.
[111] Borghouts, 1978: 43.
[112] Bardinet, 1995: 471.
[113] Nunn, 1996: 40.
[114] Lefebvre, 1958: 174.

[115] Leiden, National Museum of Antiquities, F 1895 / 5, 1, (P. Insinger); Lexa, *Papyrus Insinger IV*, 4, *OMRO* 63, 1982 and Lichtheim, 1980.
[116] Lichtheim, 1980: 190.
[117] Pinch, 1994: 117.
[118] Lichtheim, 2006: 215-216.
[119] Lichtheim, 2006: 220-222; Pinch, 1994: 127-128.
[120] Blackman, Aylward M., *The Story of King Kheops and the Magicians*, British Museum Press, London, 1988.

The *Papyri* at the Institut Français d'Archaéologie Orientale (IFAO) in Cairo include personal letters such as this *Papyrus IFAO Deir el-Medina 1*, a copy of the Teachings of Ani that has spells for good health. According to the Institute, these papyri were found in 1928 during excavations at *Deir el-Medina* but there is no certainty that they all belong to the same discovery date. The story of these papyri was reconstructed by Gardiner, Posener and Pestman; these authors thought that, in the XIXth Dynasty (13th century BC), some of the texts were copied by Kenherkhopechef, 'accountant for the project of the royal tomb'. They may have been housed at the tomb/chapel, before being moved to where they were found.[121]

Leiden Papyrus I 343+345

At Thebes several Papyri were found in the 19th century by Johann d'Anastasi,[122] which became known by this title. This fragment, Leiden I 343+345, dated from the third century AD, has essentially only magical texts[123] (spells against demons), written in Demotic. It has instructions on divination processes, some medical prescriptions such as the treatment for dog bites, extraction of venom and how to remove a bone stuck in the throat, as well as prescriptions to induce sleep, paralysis and death. On the reverse there are names of plants and animals and several prescriptions for pregnant women, gout, eye diseases and love spells.[124] It is housed at the National Museum of Amsterdam and is dated to the XVIIIth and XIXth Dynasties. It was translated by the Jesuit Egyptologist Adhémar Massart at Leiden in 1954. It is essentially about magical spells.[125] For example, a spell to repel a demon in these texts invokes divinities of a probable foreign origin (Semitic), the *samana*-demon.[126]

Schøyen Papyrus MS 2634/3

Its content refers to Epidemies II, 6:7 – 10 from Hippocrates, written in Greek, from Alexandria, dated from the end of the Second century BC to the beginning of the I BC, one fragment from which the last part of the column II, 611-22, is at Princeton University (P. Princeton AM 15960A). It is probably from the destroyed Library of Alexandria and was bought from an antiquities dealer in Cairo in 1969 by Anton Fackelmann Senior,

from Vienna. It is the first Papyrus from the Hippocratic Corpus to be published.[127] The text is divided to show correspondence and to prove that this was the way Hippocrates would have demonstrated it, because there was some rivalry among those practicing medicine in Alexandria from Ptolemaic times to Roman times. Hippocrates would have saved many medical texts from oblivion. Only this and some others give us the opportunity to have a glimpse of the ancient *corpus* before *Artemidorus Capito* is published, and before Galen interpreted these texts. They are exhibited at the BibelMuseum, Münster since 1986.[128]

Tebtunis Papyri

Written in Greek, these are housed at the Bancroft Library of Berkeley University, California.[129] There is, in the Fayoum area,[130] a crocodile cemetery where more than a thousand mummified crocodiles were found as well as a sarcophagus in 1900. These items were not only from the official excavations of the Egypt Exploration Fund in 1899/1900 and Berlin in 1902 and from the University of Milan's excavations in 1929-1936 and 1989 to present, but also many were stolen by local peasants and sold. All the Egyptian material sold at the beginning of the 20th century is now contained in private collections worldwide. As such, much of the material from Tebtunis has not been studied and those texts already studied need revising.[131]

In the remains of this temple many documents were found, from medical texts to administrative and religious texts. As a curiosity, the public toilets date from the third century AD. They had showers, stone basins and a stove to heat the bath water. In the Ptolemaic and Roman Periods there was an increase in the use of amulets, healing statues and magical papyri for personal use.

---

[121] Pestman, 1982: 155-172.

[122] Johann d'Anastasi (1780-1857), son of a Greek merchant from Damascus, who became rich supplying Napoleon's troops and later vice-consul of several Scandinavian countries. He became even richer with the commercialization of grain and using his influence during the reign of Mohammed Ali Pasha to deal on Egyptian antiquities making those getting out of the country through Alexandria. A big part of His collection was sold in 1828 and deposited at the University of Leiden. In 1885, C. Leemans finished the publication with a Latin translation of some of the texts.

[123] University College of London :
http://www.digitalegypt.ucl.ac.uk/med/healingpapyri.html

[124] Griffith, Thompson, 1904: 15-18.

[125] DuQuesne, 2002: 243.

[126] Borghouts, 1978: 18-19.

[127] M. Gronewald, *ZPE* 28, 1978: 276-277; A.E. Hanson: *SAMR* 23, 1995: 26-27; e A.E. Hanson e T. Gagos, *Well Articulated spaces, Hippocrates, Epidemics II 6, 7-22*, in *Specimina per il Corpus dei Papiri Greci de Medicina*, Firenze 1997: 117-140.

[128] The Schøyen Collection:
http://schoyencollection.com/smallercollect.htm#2634

[129] Umm el-Baragat, present name of the village next to the old Tebtunis, SW of the Fayoum, one hours drive from Medinet el-Fayoum. These texts were found at the temple dedicated to local Sobek, Soknebtunis at Tebtunis, built during the XXIIth Dynasty inhabited by Greek and Roman. Excavations were conducted during 1899/1900. This temple was built by order of Ptolemy I (305-285 BC) and later enlarged by Ptolemy XII (80-58 and 55-51 BC). Several Papyri were found, belonging to the priests of Soknebtunis near the temple. Dated approximately from the Second century AD;
http://tebtunis.berkeley.edu/collection/tebtunis.html

[130] In the fourth season of excavations from another location but also from the Greco-Roman Period, Soknopaiou Nesos, the island of the crocodile god at the Fayoum, by the team from the Centro di Studi Papirologici dell'Università di Lecce, directed by Mario Capasso and Paola Davoli, in December 2006, among other artifacts, some important papyri were found, written in Greek and Demotic:
http://tebtunis.berkeley.edu/collection/contents.html#town

[131] Abstract by Arthur Verhoogt, *New light on The Family Archive from Tebtunis*, Annual Meeting of the American Philological Association, Philadelphia, 2002.
http://www.apaclassics.org/AnnualMeeting/02mtg/abstracts/verhoogt.html

At Tebtunis, medical practice was probably undertaken by temple priests. Medical prescriptions were found in (*Tebtunis Papyrus* II 676, 677, 689) a very damaged medical treatise (*Tebtunis Papyrus* II 678), a collection of eye medicines (*Tebtunis Papyrus* 273), a fragment of *Herodotus Medicus* (*Tebtunis Papyrus* II 272) from the end of Second century AD and an illustrated herbal (*Tebtunis Papyrus* II 679), maybe the first herbal in history.[132]

Its format is according to the description from Pliny, The Elder. Each section has a preface, the name of the plant followed by a colour illustration and a description of the medical properties and medicinal preparation that can be made from it.

Some of these texts seem to have come from inside the temple, as well as some medical instruments from the same location, and this indicates that priests were actively involved in medicine at Tebtunis. Fragments from *Tebtunis Papyrus* II 275 were found in an amulet against fever in the Roman Period (I BC-IV AD). An inverted triangle is formed by a magical word repeated with successive omission of the first and the last letters, so it can be read in any direction.[133]

Yale Papyrus CtYBR 2081

Written in Greek and not yet confirmed to be a medical text, as well as being without provenance, it is housed at the Beinecke Rare Book and Manuscript Library, Yale University, New Haven, Connecticut, USA. From the Ptolemaic Period, at the end of the third century AD, also with the reference of *Yale Papyrus* 123, bought in 1966.[134]

Louvre Medical Papyrus

This is a recent acquisition from the Louvre Museum bought from the Ipsen Group.[135] It was bought by a private collector in 1953, brought to France and then sold after his death. It is thought to be the second largest medical Papyrus (after *Ebers Papyrus*) with eight sheets (seven meters), written in Hieratic (both sides) in a New Kingdom style. In the recto the first scribe (there are two) collected diagnosis and medical prescriptions; the texts are mythological in their background as the treatments are divine. It deals with several *chefut*: pustules, furuncles and abscesses, indicating how to diagnose them and presenting medical and magical prescriptions to treat them.[136]

Rubensohn Papyrus (Berlin 10456)

Housed at the Ägyptisches Museum und Papyrussammlung, Berlin[137] and written only on the recto, with prescriptions and tests to cure coughs. Its specialty is the detailed scientific language which demonstrates that, in ancient Egypt there was not only magic and superstition in the cures but also science.

Vindob Papyrus 3873

This papyrus combines Hieratic and Demotic and describes the embalmment ritual of the Apis bull in detail. The papyrus was bought at Alexandria in 1821 and is now housed at the Kunsthistorisches Museum in Vienna. It contains a description of the priests' procedures in the seventy days of mourning; his total depilation for this ceremony, with details of fasting in this period. It also describes the ritual of Apopis' death as a necessary liturgical act to this procedure. It can be included in this work as a reference to mummification and how the organs were treated.[138]

Vindob Papyrus 6257 (Crocodilopolis)

Dated from the second half of the Second century AD it does not have any magical texts but lists prescriptions from the Mediterranean area never mentioned before in Egyptian medical texts.[139]

Turin Papyrus 54003

A medical-magical papyrus, written in Hieratic, with practical medical advice and magical formulae for a good "return to life". It has also some formulae to cast away snakes[140] and protect the eyes. The spell for removing a fish spine stuck in the throat by eating bread is its *ex-libris*.[141]

Anonymus Londinensis

The *Anonymus Londinensis*[142] is based, in part, on the history of medicine written in the 4th century BC by Meno, a disciple of Aristotle. Philolaus of Croton

---

and also a lecturer on Egyptian Archaeology at the École du Louvre says that the papyrus is being studied following this exhibition. The Project will last three years (private e-mail and at an interview to the *Le Monde* in June, 7, 2007: http://www.lemonde.fr/web/video/0,47-0@2-3246,54-919933@51-919937,0.html.

[137] Rubensohn worked at Abusir in 1908 collecting papyri found in Alexandria.

[138] *The Apis Embalming Ritual, P. Vindob 3873*, Orientalia Lovaniensia Analecta, 50, 1992.

[139] Nunn, 1996: 41.

[140] Borghouts, 1978: 91.

[141] Borghouts, 1978: 23 and http://digilander.libero.it/Egitto_Antico/SDP_CompendioPapiri3.pdf. Publicado por Roccati, A., *Papyrus ieratico n. 54003,. Estratti magici e rituali del Primo Medio Regno*, Turin 1970.

[142] Diels, Hermann, *Anonymi Londinensis ex Aristotelis Iatricis Menoniis et aliis medicis eclogae / edidit Hermannus Diels*, Berlin, Kingmer, 1893, [xviii]-76 p. Coll. CAG, Supl. 3.1 [231]; *Anonymus Londinensis*, University Press, Cambridge, 1947.

---

[132] Tebtunis Papyri: http://tebtunis.berkeley.edu/collection/imagesindex.html

[133] http://tebtunis.berkeley.edu/collection/imagesindex.html

[134] Beinecke Rare Book and Manuscript Library, Papyrus Collection: http://beinecke.library.yale.edu/papyrus/SearchExec.asp

[135]http://web.culture.fr/culture/actualites/dossiers-presse/papyrus2007/dp-papyrus.pdf

[136] Shown at a recent exhibition at the Louvre, from June 6 to August 6, 2007, about the medical arts in ancient Egypt. Marc Étienne, curator of this exhibition, from the ancient Egyptian Art Department at the Louvre

explained disease considering three factors: bile, blood and phlegm.[143] It is a long papyrus about the execration theory. It is the longest Greek papyrus found so far, written in the Second century AD. Classified as BM 137, it has a Latin introduction, and a Greek text with notes.[144]

Louvre Papyrus E 4864

It has a small medical text in the verso. Dated from the XVIIIth Dynasty, c. 1400 BC[145]

Borgia Papyrus

Forty to fifty Greek papyri were found buried in a vase in the Fayoum area, where Ptolemy Philadelphos had his Greek veterans. One of these papyri was bought and ended up in the hands of Cardinal Stefano Borgia in 1778; the others were destroyed as they were thought to be worthless. *Borgia Papyrus* (3.5 m) was published ten years after and records the forced labour of peasants (a long list of names) building the Nile embankment at Tebtunis, between 192 and 193 AD.[146]

Chassinat *IFAO* Coptic *Papyrus*

This Coptic manuscript from the 9th century AD was found by peasants at Meshaikh[147] and brought by Bouriant[148] to the Institut Français D'Archéologie Orientale in the Cairo Library, in the winter of 1892-83.[149] The text shows that scientific tradition was not lost between the pagan period and the Christian era in Egypt; native (ancient Egyptian), Greek and Christian traditions were combined.

Arab rulers of medieval Egypt had much confidence in Christian doctors and their work was translated from Coptic to Arabic, although there are few Coptic texts of this type known today, written in Sahidic,[150] possibly due to material deterioration. Another problem is the

identification of the ingredients used in prescriptions; this text has some symbols from alchemy and pharmacy.[151] It has prescriptions for eye and skin diseases that are copies from Old Kingdom texts.[152]

There are other papyri in existence which are relevant in the study of medicine in ancient Egypt; some Greek fragments of medical texts are spread worldwide in different institutions. These are mentioned next with brief references as found in the researched bibliography:

Physiology Treaty in three fragments written in the first century BC; *Rylands Papyrus* 1.21 (John Rylands Library, Manchester, UK); *Berliner Papyrus Klassikertexte* BKT 3.10-19 (inv. 9770) (Staatliche Museen zu Berlin); *Kingnach Papyrus* 1.2, *Papyrus Sorbonne* (inv.2011) (Institut de Papyrologie de la Sorbonne, Université de Paris).[153]

An ophthalmology treaty in four fragments, from the first half of the Second century BC; *Rylands Papyrus* 1.39 (John Rylands Library, Manchester, UK); *Grenfell Papyrus* 2.7b (Bodleian Library Greek E.63 (P), (Oxford); *Heidelberg Papyrus* inv. 401 (Heidelberg); *Hibeh Papyrus* 2.190 (BM 2963) (British Museum).[154]

Ophthalmology questionnaire written in the Second century AD; *Ross Georg Papyrus* 1.20 (P. Golenischeff, Museum of Fine Arts, Moscow).[155]

Scroll with ophthalmology prescriptions with notes on the verso; *Argentoratenses Graecae Papyri* (Programm, Rostock 1901) 8-12 (*Papyrus Strasburg* inv.Gr.1, centuries III-IV).[156]

Oxyrhynchus Papyrus 1384

From the 5th century AD, it has three medical prescriptions for purge, a drink to ease urine, for wounds and two healing legends.[157]

1.11. Ostraca

Besides Papyri with relevance to the study of medicine and health in ancient Egypt, there are ostraca with therapeutical inscriptions that are important to mention:[158]

---

[143] Huffman, 1993: 88; Stanford University, California, USA: http://plato.stanford.edu/entries/philolaus/
Paris: http://callimac.vjf.cnrs.fr/RSPA/References/References_A.html#P_91
[144] Centre national de la recherche scientifique, http://callimac.vjf.cnrs.fr/RSPA/References/References_A.html#P_91
[145] University College London: http://www.digitalegypt.ucl.ac.uk/literature/loyalist/sources.html
[146] Head, Peter, Tyndale House, Residential Centre for Biblical Studies, Cambridge: http://www.tyndale.cam.ac.uk/Tyndale/staff/Head/NT&Pap1.htm; Bromiley, 1995: 652.
[147] Schoff, 1925: 76.
[148] Bouriant, U., *Fragment d'un livre de médecine en copte thébain*, *Comptes rendus de l'Académie des Inscriptions et Belles-Lettres*, série 4, 15, 1887 : 374-379.
[149] Chassinat, 1921.
[150] Probable origins of this name: from *Sayhad*, name given by the Islamic geographers to the Ramlat al-Sab'atayn desert, or from the Arabic *as-Said* (Upper Egypt). The Bohairic, spoken in the Lower Egypt, is the present liturgical Coptic language used. Other dialects: Fayoumic, Akhimic and Licopolitan. An interesting work done on this matter: Azevedo, Joaquim, *A Simplified Coptic Dictionary (Sahidic Dialect)*, Centro de Pesquisa de Literatura Bíblica, Tools for Exegesis, CePLiB 1, Seminário Adventista Latino-Americano de Teologia, 2001.

[151] Chassinat, 1921.
[152] Some notes were given to me by Nicole Hansen from the Oriental Institute of Chicago which I thank her for.
[153] Pack, 1965: 126 (2346). In this work by Roger Pack there are approximately a hundred references to fragments with medical texts dated from between the Second century BC (2344), and the 4th century AD (several) between pages 126-128. Many are surely re-editions from ancient Egyptian texts, but there is no scientific evidence of that yet.
[154] Pack, 1965: 37 (342).
[155] Pack, 1965: 126 (2343).
[156] Pack, 1965: 127 (2380).
[157] Meyer, 1994: 31.
[158] Medizinische Ostraka des Alten Ägyptens: http://www.medizinische-papyri.de/html/medizinische_ostraka.html

Ostracon Berlin 5570 – Three prescriptions for a non specified disease

Ostracon Deir el-Medina 1062 – Proverb and magical prescription for an eye disease
Ostracon Deir el-Medina 1091 – Two prescriptions for skin treatment
Ostracon Deir el-Medina 1216 – Magic for abdominal disease
Ostracon Deir el-Medina 1242 – Incomplete prescription for a non specified disease
Ostracon Deir el-Medina 1414 – Incomplete prescription for a non specified disease

Ostracon Leiden 334 – Prescription for a non specified disease
Ostracon Louvre 3255 – Prescription for a non specified ear disease by fumigation[159]
Ostracon London 297 – Prescription for a non specified disease
Ostracon Turin 57104 – List of body parts[160]
Ostracon from Thebes at the Royal Ontario Museum – A disease prevention[161]
Ostracon Bodleian Greek 923 – Colirium prescription (eye).[162]

1.12. Mummies

"...In fact, almost every mummy has a unique scent..."[163]
The first report of radiological research done on an Egyptian mummy was published by Petrie in 1898.[164]

Our present knowledge of disease and health patterns has been growing with the scientific study of Egyptian mummified bodies, either to detect traces of trauma and diseases or to examine parasites in the sarcophagi, as well as the inscriptions on the sarcophagi, linen bandages and amulets that cover the mummies.

The "covering bandage of the doctor's equipment", the ḥ3yt nt ḥn swnw, used the ḥ3yt, a type of bandage used by the priest who performs the mummification and also by the doctor.[165]

The mummification started to happen naturally in the bodies left in the Egyptian underground; hot and dry,

being "hot-dried" by the sun; the very hot climate favours the drying out of the body so keeping it in a good state of preservation. It is almost impossible today to try to pinpoint the date when mummification became a common mortuary practice, but there is suggestion that it must have begun after visualizing how the bodies left in the desert were naturally preserved,[166] around the IV Dynasty (2600 BC). Records of mummification practice are only recorded in the New Kingdom but the oldest mummies found to date are those from the Pre-Dynastic cemetery at Hierakonpolis, HK43 in Upper Egypt, Wadi Khamsini. Research in this cemetery began in 1996 and after five seasons, 260 graves were found containing close to 300 individuals, probably workers from the Naqada Period, IIA-C (3600-3400 BC).[167]

3.1. Origin of the word and analysis formula; "mummy powder" as medicine

"...mummy: human remains, resin, wrapping, and all..."
[168]

So, where did this word come from, so connected to ancient Egypt?

The word ⟨hieroglyphs⟩, sśḥ,[169] (sarcophagus,

⟨hieroglyphs⟩ wi[170]), meant "mummy" in ancient Egyptian, but also bitumen or "bitumen material", as a reference to the black colour of the Egyptian mummified bodies when unwrapped, this comes from the medieval Latin word mumia,[171] loaned from then Arabic mūmiyyah, مومية, which means bitumen. According to Abdel Latif, an Arab doctor of the 12th century, who travelled to Egypt, this substance would have its origin in the Persian mūmiya, bitumen, as this was flowing down from a mountain and, mixing with ice turned into water; thus originated, this substance was thought to have medicinal properties.[172]

From the 12th century onwards, travellers going to Persia spoke about mummies with miraculous properties, healing wounds instantly and mending broken bones. When Persian travellers went to Egypt and saw the mummified bodies covered by a black substance similar to mummia, they misinterpreted it and mummia became the name for the body covering and the body itself. Then, a real 'hunt for Egyptian mummies' began. The highest selling point in history would have been in the Middle Ages and again in the XVIIth and XVIIIth centuries. Many boticaries diluted this substance in wine, honey or water. In some cases the substance was not powdered, but as pieces of the body or in a paste.

---

[159] Jonckheere, Frans, L'Ostracon médical du Louvre, Sudhoffs Archiv für Geschichte der Medizin und der Naturwissenschaften, Wiesbaden, 37,3/4, 278-282, November 1953; CdE XXIX, N° 57, 53-56, 1954.
[160] Halioua, 2005.
[161] Ostracon with a spell to prevent the attack of a demon. The body parts where this demon should not "come in" are described. Theban ostraca: Edited from the originals, now mainly in the Royal Ontario Museum of Archaeology, Toronto, and the Bodleian Library, Oxford, 1913..According to the Griffith Institute, Oxford, ?50.28-9.
[162] (Pack 2427), discovered at Thebes and written in the 4th century AD, at the Ashmolean Museum, Oxford.
[163] David, 2000: 12
[164] Petrie, W.M.F., Deshasheh, 1897, Fifteenth memoir of the Egypt Exploration Fund, London, 1898.
[165] Győry, 2006: 1.

[166] Moodie, 1931: 19.
[167] Hierakonpolis, http://www.hierakonpolis.org/site/hk43.html
[168] David, 2000: 40.
[169] Faulkner, 2006: 215.
[170] Faulkner, 2006: 56.
[171] It meant, in Latin, to lie down in aromatic resins, one of the last stage of mummification procedures; Ebeid, 1999:422.
[172] David and Tapp, 1993: 37.

A surgeon from Bretagne, Ambrósio Paré (1510-1590), was one of the first to criticize this medicine. His criticism was based upon what was told to him by Gui de la Fontaine, the kings' doctor from Navarra. He would have travelled in 1564 to Alexandria. There he knew about a Jew who dealt in mummies and this one confessed that the bodies were not older than four years.[173]

In 1658, Sir Thomas Browne, a philosopher, referred to mummy powder as: "mummy is become merchandise, *mizraim* cures wounds and pharaoh is sold for *balsama*" and maybe before the 12th century, doctors prescribed this medicine to their patients.[174]

The work *Rates for the Custom House in London* mentions "crushed mummy"; and in 1657 the work *The Physical Dictionary* contained the definition: "Mummy, something like resin that is sold in boticaries; some say it is extracted from ancient tombs". In Spain, Benito Jerónimo Feijoo (1676-1764), a Benedictine monk, Professor of Theology and Sacred Scriptures and a big defender of ascetic medicine, was a strong critic of mummy powder.[175]

The physician John Hall is referenced as having used this "medicine" in two of his patients:

"William Fortesque, aged 20, was troubled with the Falling-sickness, by consent from the Stomach, as also hypochondriac melancholy, with a depravation of both Sense and Motion of the two middle Fingers of the Right-hand" (p.50, observation XXIX); Melvin Earles' comment: In this condition the patient exhibits a morbid preoccupation with ill health. [...] at the onset of a fit the patient was made to inhale a vapour formed by burning a mixture of the aromatic resin benzoin, powdered mummy, black pitch and juice of rue." (p. 55); Patient Mr. P. (Observation XIII, page. 196) was "afflicted with a Flux of Semen, and Night-pollutions, by which he was much weakened". He had a pill prescribed with gum Arabic, tragacanth gum, Armenian bole, carabe (amber), mummy powder and *Mandibule Lucii piscis*[176] or jaw of pike, all items believed to hinder or stop fluxes. Melvin Earles comments in a footnote on p.197: "Mummy was included in the London Pharmacopoeia of 1618. It was said to pierce all parts, restore wasted limbs, cure consumptions and ulcers, hinder blood coagulation and stop fluxes. A shortage of the genuine article resulted in recipes for making artificial mummy from the newly dead" (cf. Webster's White Devil, I.1.17ff) "

In 1833, Thomas J. Pettigrew, later known as 'Mummy Pettigrew', bought a mummy for 23 pounds when Henry Salt's collection was put to sale and he unwrapped it at the Charing Cross Hospital in London, where he was a Professor of Anatomy. In 1834, he presented a mummy to the Royal College of Surgeons and in the next twenty years, it was one mummy after another, always with a full house. In 1852 Pettigrew mummified the body of Alexander, the tenth Duke of Hamilton, by his own request.[177] The mummy was preserved in an Egyptian sarcophagus in the Duke's mausoleum at his property; he was a traveller to Egypt and a collector for the British Museum and for himself.

Sir Marc Armand Ruffer (1859-1917), pioneer of paleopathology, developed a formula to study the mummified tissues, softening them with alcohol and 5% of sodium bicarbonate.[178] Ruffer says: "...Indeed, it is a striking fact that up to the present I have never found bitumen in any mummy, even in those of the Ptolemaic period. (March 1911). "[179]

Nevertheless we went from mummy powder as a medicine to biochemical research in mummies for scientific purposes. The inorganic substances used in mummification, according to Alfred Lucas,[180] would have been natron and salt. In the resinous material from the mummies' bandages traces of natron are also found.

3.2. Ancient Egyptian words related to mummification:

-linen bandage[181] *wt*

-embalming action[182] *sdwh*

- linen bandage[183] *swdwd*

-natron[184] *hsmn*

-place of embalming,[185] *wt*

-embalmer, bandager,[186] *wt*

-mummy sarcophagus,[187] *wi*

[173] Jofre, 2004:1.
[174] Ebeid, 1999: 423; David e Tapp, 1993: 11.
[175] In *El Teatro Crítico Universal o Discursos varios en todo género de materias para desengaño de errores comunes*, tomo 4° Discurso 12: 25, Feijoo speaks of mummy powder:
http://filosofia.org/bjf/bjft412.htm#t41220; Jofre, 2004:
http://www.Egyptlogia.com/content/view/565/91/
[176] Lúcio (peixe de rio): http://web2.bium.univ-paris5.fr/livanc/?cote=00216x04&p=490&do=page

[177] Spindler, 1996: 5.
[178] Ruffer, 1921: 64.
[179] Ruffer, 1921: 21, 54.
[180] Lucas, 1926: 110-125.
[181] Faulkner, 2006: 71.
[182] Faulkner, 2006: 256.
[183] Faulkner, 2006: 218.
[184] Faulkner, 2006: 178.
[185] Faulkner, 2006: 71. There is an alabaster embalming table, probably from the IIIrd Dynasty, c. 2650 BC, found in the enclosure of Djoser's pyramid, in Saqqara.
[186] Faulkner, 2006: 71.

-priest (pure),[188] $w'b$

-purification tent[189] where the process of mummification began and the body was cleansed. Next to water (river or channel) ibw

-place of embalming (temporary adobe buildings);[190] kitchen or refectory close to tomb, where the body was taken to after being purified. The *uabt neb ut* would have been the embalming place to prepare the bodies of highest ranked individuals; it was next to the adjacent tomb wt

Ex: tomb of Kai, priest of the kings Khufu and Khafre in Giza.[191]

-"beautiful house"; funerary house[192] where the body was eviscerated, dissected, embalmed, bandaged with linen, soaked in resin and put into the sarcophagus, $pr\ nfr$

3. 3. Process of mummification summarily described

The preservation of the human body after death was an essential pre-condition to extend the existence of that person. This ancient Egyptian thought is probably based on the Myth of Osiris, the first mummy, made by Isis. The written literature on this subject is detached from Classical authors such as Herodotus (deceased c. 406 BC) and Diodorus Sículus, who died about 440 years later. Their descriptions may not represent exactly the practices undertaken over a thousand years before their existence, when embalming deceased people was common in ancient Egypt.

The Embalming Ritual is described in two Papyri, probably copied from the same ancient source, dating from the Greco-Roman period, and housed in Cairo: *Papyrus Bulaq* 3, and at the Louvre, *Papyrus* 5158.[193] In the latter, the embalming is said to begin only four days after death and the linen bandaging 46 days after, so 42 days are left for the rituals. They used incense oil[194] and the used resin worked as glue so it should be sticky to make the linen bandages adhere well.

There are also references to this ritual in the *Rhind Papyrus* (c. 1650 BC, where the scribe Ahmes[195] states that he copied this text from an ancient document from the XIIth Dynasty, c. 1800 BC), housed today at the British Museum.

The study of the process of mummification and its procedures has been providing new data about the treatment that was given to the bodies of the deceased and, even better for this field of research, information on diseases, diet, daily life and family interactions in ancient Egypt.

Regarding Examples of the mummification of children and infants are scarce from the beginning of the 20th century.[196]

A detail: the Seven Sacred Oils mentioned in the Opening of the Mouth Ritual in the Pyramid Texts. These oils were also used for medicinal purposes, perfumes and massages, as well as for kitchen use and home lighting. There are examples of little tables with seven cavities for the Seven Oils with hieroglyphic inscriptions such as the one found in the tomb of Qar, a physician from Saqqara.[197]

At the centennial commemorations of the Egyptian Museum in Cairo, one of these tables on display contained the following inscriptions, from left to right: *Sethh-heb*, perfume used in the festival; *sefeth*, unknown; *hekenu*, from the first class resins *ab* and *antiu*, to annoint the divine members (formula at the wall from the temple of Edfu next to the king' statue); *nemu*, unknown; *tUžst*, unknown; *ha-ach* (from the *Conifera* tree, *Albies alba*, cedar tree); *haentehennu* (from Libia).[198]

More examples of these tables can be seen at the British Museum (6122, 6123, 29421).[199]

Mummification was a religious practice but it can also be seen as a precocious scientific activity that gave the embalmers much knowledge about the human body.[200] The techniques used in the analysis of Egyptian mummified bodies have developed from the X-rays to endoscopies (a different equipment used in mummies from the one used in living people as mummies have no fluids), to CAT scans (computerized axial tomography), and more recently to DNA studies. In 1985 Svante Pääbo, a Swedish molecular biologist from the Uppsala

---

[187] Faulkner, 2006: 56.

[188] Faulkner, 2006: 57.

[189] Faulkner, 2006: 15.

[190] Faulkner, 2006: 71.

[191] Zahi A. Hawass, *Opening the Lost Tombs: Live from Egypt*, first TV documentary about an Egyptian excavation for the Western world, made by FOX, 1999.

[192] Faulkner, 2006: 89.

[193] Colombini, 2000: 19; Brier, Wade, 2001: 1.

[194] Fragranced resins, *Boswellia* africana and arabica was used in the embalmment, as well as the Sudanese *Boswellia papyrifera Rich*; Liber Herbarum. http://www.liberherbarum.com/Index.htm

[195] Or Ahmose, that lived in the Second Intermediate Period. University of Illinois at Urbana-Champaign, USA: http://archive.ncsa.uiuc.edu/Cyberia/VideoTestbed/Projects/Mummy/egypt.html

[196] Moodie, 1931: 19.

[197] http://www.osirisnet.net/docu/centennial/centennial.htm

[198] Budge, 1996: 30;
http://www.osirisnet.net/docu/centennial/centennial.htm

[199] Budge, 1996: 30.

[200] Fleming, Fishman, O'Connor, Silverman, 1980.

University, extracted DNA from an Egyptian mummy, although his results cannot be reproduced.[201]

Herodotus' reports continue, nevertheless, to be the most complete.[202] The embalmer extracted the brain out through the nasal cavity with the help of a hook, breaking the ethmoid bone[203] and twisting the hook (usually a bronze one) to liquefy the brain matter and ease it out through the nostrils. Next, the cavity was filled with resin, bitumen and unguents. A spoon was used to do this, covering the cavities (inside of the skull and nostrils). As they considered the heart the centre for emotions and thinking, the brain matter was discarded as they found no useful or sacred meaning for that. From the IVth Dynasty onwards evisceration was practised making a left incision on the abdomen, with an obsidian knife[204] and afterwards removing the organs by hand.

There are cases found were evisceration was not practised and others where[205] an evisceration *per anum* was performed.[206] In the precise spot where the incision was made, there is sometimes found a Horus eye drawn as to protect the body entry/exit.[207]

The ancient Egyptian divided the body in 36 parts; each one ruled by either a dean or a demon, who presided over the triple divisions from the twelve signs of the Zodiac. A sort of 'theological anatomy' was made by Champollion, based upon the 'great funereal Ritual · or book of Manifestations'.[208]

The deceased body rested in natron for different periods, according to the financial possibilities of his/her family; the wealthiest for seventy days (observing the Sirius star)[209] and the bandages were changed as they became soaked in body fluids. The ancient Egyptians used natron as a drying agent to accentuate natural desiccation and the quantities used and its quality visibly affected the state of preservation of the bodies, as seen in mummified examples. Small quantities or frequent and repeated use of the same batch reduced the effectiveness. Natron is a chemical mixture of sodium carbonate and bicarbonate[210] found in natural deposits in Egypt, in the Wadi Natrun area its composition varies with different amounts of

sodium carbonate, chlorate and sulphate. It also contains clay and calcium carbonate in lesser quantities. The impurities of sodium chlorate and sulphate[211] affect the efficacy of its use.[212]

The practice of leaving the organs inside the body, wrapped in linen bandages and soaked in resins, was discontinued from the Greco-Roman period onwards. After the desiccation by natron period the last stage of mummification took place; enclosing the body in a sarcophagus. The skin was soaked in melted resin, covering it, which strengthened it and helped close pores in the skin so humidity would not damage the body.[213]

The heart was wrapped and protected by amulets, usually a stone scarab inscribed with chapter 30 from The Book of The Dead, requesting a favourable testimony at the Final Judgement. The body was then completely wrapped, sometimes with amulets, and amulet-papyri,[214] magical spells written in individual rolls of papyrus; some were used also in life by its owner, and then carried with them on this final journey.[215]

Papyrus Heidelberg G1359, as it was folded, suggests it could have been used as such;[216] also *Papyrus Michigan* 3023a was rolled and bent to serve as an amulet.[217]

Amulets are, in most cases, elements of funerary purpose but, both literature and archaeology have shown that its protective function was also used in life with great significance.

The organs that were considered to be essential in another life were preserved, in canopic vases.[218] There were four vases and their lids/heads were represented by the four sons of Horus: Duamutef, Imsety, Kebehsenuef and Hapi, and, protecting those, four different deities, as shown below. There are theories regarding Imsety: could she be a female element and not a hermaphrodite as other theories state because she is fair skinned and the face features are female? There are representations of the late period that show Imsety as a woman.[219] This is a

[201] David, 2000: 150.

[202] David, Tapp, 1993: 42.

[203] David, 2000: 70.

[204] Sharp knife from Ethiopia: Ebeid, 1999: 427; David, Tapp, 1993: 44; obsidian is a volcanic glass from outside Egypt (Ethiopia) documented in several collections (different knifes) Manchester Museum (a piece of obsidian), Petrie Museum, London.

[205] Ebeid, 1999: 431,434.

[206] David, Tapp, 1993: 44.

[207] Pettigrew, 1838: 11.

[208] Pettigrew, 1838: 12: "...This is expressed, on various mummy-cases, in hieroglyphics.
characters ; and may we not in this trace the first attempt to assign the different parts of the body to the several planets...", http://www.archive.org/stream/biographicalmemo01pettuoft/biographicalmemo01pettuoft_djvu.txt

[209] Ebeid, 1999: 443.

[210] Ebeid, 1999: 437-442. Sodium carbonate (Na_2CO_3). Sodium bicarbonate ($NaHCO_3$).

[211] Sodium chlorate (NaCl). Sodium sulfate (Na_2SO_4).

[212] David, Tapp, 1993: 43. Melanie Sapsford is a specialist on these matters, finishing a PhD on chemicals of ancient Egypt at the DCMT Cranfield University, Royal Military College of Science.

[213] Luxor Mummification Museum Catalogue, 1997

[214] Oracle or amulet-papyri.

[215] Pinch, 1994: 116-117; Fleming, Fishman, O'Connor, Silverman, 1980: 22. An example from the Louvre, Paris, n.3233, has a short magical formula with prophylactic drawings to protect a child, casting away evils from the year and praying to Sekhmet among other deities; Goyon, 1977: 45-54.

[216] Meyer e Smith, 1994: 30.

[217] Meyer e Smith, 1994: 250.

[218] The origin of the name comes from the town of Canopus, West of Alexandria, near modern Abu Qir. Canopus was revered as a form of Osiris at Abu Qir symbolized by a globular vase, Aufderheide, 2003: 257.

[219] "...a young woman dressed in green kneels in front of an anthropomorphic deity (Imsety?)..", http://www.virtual-egyptian-Museumm.org/Collection/FullVisit/Collection.FullVisit-FR.html

probability as her name ends with a *t* (sign for female in hieroglyphic writing).

Until the 4th century AD, mummification was frequent but then it started to decline as the growing Christian community did not request this ritual. In the 5th century mummies were no longer made and so this cultural element of Egypt was lost.[220]

The lungs, intestines, stomach and liver were treated with resins and bandaged to stay in their canopic vases. But in other cases mummies have these organs placed again inside the body *in situ*.[221] A change of time, a change of will...

Protective deity	Goddess	Head	Organ	Cardinal
Imseti	Isis	Human	Liver	Sul
Hapi	Nephtys	Babuíno	Lungs	Norte
Duamutef	Neit	Chacal	Stomach	Este
Kebehsenuef	Serket	Falcão	Intestines	Oeste

3. 4. Example cases of analyzed Egyptian mummies

A small introductory note regarding the analysis of mummified bodies in Egypt is given by Denon: "the number of bodies not bandaged showed that circumcision was known and generally practised, that depilation in women was not performed as today, that their hair was straight and long..."[222] We can conclude from this that, in 1798 female depilation was common although not as usual as today and that the long and straight hair seen by Denon in these mummies would have been natural hair and not wigs.

With the discovery of X-rays by Roentgen in 1895 and subsequent development of radiology, a fundamental step was made in medical diagnostics. The identification of DNA, developed in 1985, was improved in 1991 with the discovery of the Polymerase Chain Reaction (PCR), where DNA can be cloned to produce multiple copies of specific regions which was the next step to improve biomedical research. This method also shows genetic correlation between individuals (family ties).

The digital genetic imprint of an individual is influenced by the genes of his/her relatives, being mitochondrial DNA inherited from the mother, and nuclear DNA from the two breeders, a much more difficult sample to get.[223]
The limitations in DNA studies result from its decomposition with time, when the sequences are broken, and this can bring false results.[224]

In the mummy desiccation process by natron, depilation is forced and nails are destroyed. A substance that included potassium (K), phosphorus (P), iron (Fe), magnesium (Mn) and zinc (Zn), was then used for cosmetic purposes to rebuild the nails or in another option, they were sewn with thread.

The participating teams in projects like these, that analyze mummies, are composed of several professional specialists Egyptologists, radiologists, anthropologists, paleobotanists, entomologists, chemists, histopatologists, computer technicians, textiles' conservators and geneticists. This is not a work to be done by one individual only and so it is justifiable to put together theory with practice; letters and sciences, researchers, professors and students. The examination must be followed by autopsy, if possible, to confirm the results. The following examples are brief summaries of studies on mummies found to have diseases.

TT99 –Sennefer Tomb in Western Thebes

Two cases are to be mentioned regarding the mummies found in this tomb. The first is a male skull with several holes of different sizes but all with typical characteristics of metastasis from a meningioma which spread through the whole body.[225] A small number of cancers spread from soft tissue to bone[226] and in a man the most probable cause could be lung cancer. The incidence of lung cancer in ancient Egypt is relatively low and is only related to smoking habits in the modern world; a case of bone cancer in Antiquity is of considerable importance. A study of this tombs' material, published in the *Journal of Neurology, Neurosurgery and Psychiatry* in 2001, reveals that two of the mummies suffered from Parry-Romberg syndrome. This syndrome is a progressive disease in which bones from the sides of the face disintegrate and this can lead to epilepsy. Three of the skulls had the eyes turned inside, an abnormality connected to the central nervous system. One of the mummies could have suffered from *diabetes mellitus*; because it showed oval eyes (corectopy) and 24% of diabetic people suffer from corectopy. According to the researchers of this tomb, paleoneurology (paleontology and neurology) enables the research for neurological diseases in the mummified Egyptian bodies, dead over two thousand years ago, even when there are no traces of the neurological system to be analyzed.[227]

Tomb TT320 or Deir el-Bahari DB320

---

[220] Fleming, Fishman, O'Connor, Silverman, 1980: 50.

[221] Pettigrew, 1838: 11.

[222] Denon, 2004: 270.

[223] Prof. Eugénia Cunha in a session of Forensic Anthropology at the Instituto de Medicina Legal de Lisboa (Forensic Institute), February 2007.

[224]*Secrets of the Ancient World Revealed Through DNA*, presentation from Scott Woodward, professor of Microbiology at Brigham Young

University in April, 2001 summarized by Judy Greenfield in *Journal of The Egyptian Study Society*, volume 12 no. 1, 2001:.1-4. http://www.egyptologyonline.com/using_dna.htm

[225] Cancer that originates in the *dura mater*, the bony covering of the skull, that spreads and grows in diameter. It can cause pressure in the skull and cause death. In this case the tumor was small and it was thought not to be the primary cause of death. http://www.newton.cam.ac.uk/egypt/tt99/report02/index.html

[226] Campillo, 2001: 150; 279; Ruffer, 1921: 50.

[227] Nigel and Helen Strudwick, Rosalind Janssen, Bridget Leach, Rita Lucarelli, Lynn Meskell: http://www.newton.cam.ac.uk/egypt/tt99/reports.html

From the discoveries made in 1881, revealed after the confession of the Rassul brothers, tomb thieves, the bodies found were brought from different graves in the reigns of Psusennes I (1039-991 BC) and Sheshonk I (945-924 BC.). The 36 mummies were studied and numbered in ten days by Tony Waldron in 1998 and then by Helen and Nigel Strudwick in 2001 and again by Tony Waldron in 2002. The mummified Egyptians found in this tomb seem to have all died of natural causes or by wounds inflicted in battle. Some are of curious importance, n. 61051,[227] Seqenenre-Taa II, who died in battle against the Hyksos.[228] He seems to have been stabbed behind one ear because he shows a crushed face, probably with a mace, deep wounds below the right eye and traces of an axe wound in his forehead.[229] Salima Ikram and Aidan Dodson state that the wound behind the ear can be *pre-mortem*. N. 61066,[230] Tutmes II, son of Tutmes I and queen Mutnofret, husband of Hatshepsut and father of Neferure, was almost bald and his face was much wrinkled, so his death must have occurred after 30 years of age. He was unwrapped by Gaston Maspero in 1886, and then analysed by Grafton Elliot Smith in 1906.[231] Both Maspero and Smith, Ikram e Dodson[232] point to his skin[233] as having symptoms of an unknown disease because of the numerous ecchymosis and these might have been the cause of death. Smith, nevertheless states that his skin eruptions might also have been *post mortem* as a reaction from the tissue to embalming materials.

N. 61077,[234] Seti I, son of Ramesses I and Tiy; his mummy shows that he must have lived until his sixties and that he might have died of an ear infection. In 2006 the Centre for Egyptological Studies of the Russian Academy of Sciences and the Egyptology and Coptology Institute from Westfälische Wilhelms-Universität, Münster conducted their fifth and last season so far, at the necropolis of Deir el-Banat, where they found, in 2006 alone, 74 bodies that were examined.[235]

To further research on this matter it is necessary to mention that the KNH Centre from Manchester, created in 1997, has a database containing information on mummy samples provided from institutions around the world that are housed in a mummy databank.

The table below is an example list containing known examinations on Egyptian mummies undertaken to date:

Authors	Date and tests conducted
Augustus Bozzi Granville,[236] London	1820 Female, XXVII Dynasty, Dissected
T. J. Pettigrew, Jersey island Museum, UK[237]	1837 Peteviltiomes Macroscopical exam
Project Anubis (Museums of Italy)[238]	1884-1979 101 mummies Florence mummies and their paleopathological conditions were studied between 1999-2000[239]
Leeds Philosophical and Literary Society, Leeds, UK[240] Manchester Mummy Project	1828 NatsefAmun Dissected, chemical analysis, anatomical study 1990 Radiology, CAT, endoscopy, histology, serology and dental exam
Grafton Elliot Smith[241] Egyptian Museum Cairo	1890-1912 49 mummies
Museum Egyptian do Cairo	1903 Tutmes III - *CG61068*
Hancock Museum, Newcastle	1830, 1964 Baketnethor macroscopical observation, radiology

---

[227] Cairo Museumm *CG61056*.

[228] Fleming, Fishman, O'Connor, Silverman, 1980: 27.

[229] A recent X-ray, shows the bone around the point of trauma to have traces of remodelling, so, the trauma must have occurred *pre mortem*, some months before death: Fleming, Fishman, O'Connor, Silverman, 1980: 27.

[230] Cairo Museumm *CG61066*

[231] Smith, 1912: 1-6, 28-31, 57-59.

[232] Ikram, Dodson, *Mummy in Ancient Egypt: Equipping the Dead for Eternity*, Thames & Hudson, June 1998

[233] Small report on Tutmes II mummy:
http://members.tripod.com/anubis4_2000/mummypages1/Aeighteen.htm#Tuthmosis II

[234] Emory University's Michael C. Carlos Museum, 1999.1.4.

[235] The Centre for Egyptological Studies of the Russian Academy of Sciences was created in November, 1999. At its origin was the Department of Egyptology from the Oriental Studies Institute of the Russian Academy of Sciences, existing since 1992. Its deputy director, Alexey Krol, has been in touch with the author of this work providing information; http://www.cesras.ru/eng/arch/db/rep.html
http://www.cesras.ru/eng/arch/tt320/index.htm;http://www.cesras.ru/eng/arch/tt320/rep.htm;
http://members.tripod.com/anubis4_2000/mummypages1/Aeighteen.htm#Tuthmosis II

---

[236] Sakula, 1983: 876– 882. As presented at the ARCE of Seattle, Washington, USA: *The Mummy in the Drawing Room* by W. Benson Harer, Jr, March, 8th, 2003 at the Seattle Art Museum, this mummy was a *souvenir* bought for four dollars at Thebes by Sir Archibald Edmonston, the first European to visit the Western Oasis in Egypt he was called to assist Edmonston in 1824. They made the first scientific autopsy of the mummy, concluding that she must have died of ovarian cancer. After numerous pages on bandages, and 'racial issues' Granville wrote some paragraphs on a probable ovarian cyst: "The disease which appears to have destroyed her was ovarian dropsy attended with structural derangement of the uterine system generally." At the presentation, Harer, describes a modern autopsy telling a different story; Seattle Art Museum:
http://www.seattleartMuseumm.org/calendar/eventDetail.asp?eventID=4154&month=2&day=8&year=2003&sxID=&WHEN=&sxTitle=

[237] Pettigrew, 1838: 10-14.

[238] http://www.egittologia.unipi.it/project.htm

[239] Fornaciari, 2001: 17

[240] David e Tapp, 1993: 9.

[241] Smith, 1912: 1-6, 28-31, 57-59. In 1900, Smith was Chair of Anatomy at the Government School of Medicine in Cairo, until 1909. He was interested in preserving brains recovered from El-Amrah conducting research on findings at this archaeological site. In 1907, he was the Anatomical Counsellor for the Archaeological Census of Nubia financed by the Royal Society. His research on this project analysed thousands of skeletons excavated before the building of the Big Aswan Dam: Minnesota State University,
http://www.mnsu.edu/eMuseumm/information/biography/pqrst/smith_grafton.html

Authors	Date and tests conducted
Manchester Mummy Research Project, KNH Centre, Manchester, UK[243]	1908 Margaret Murray The Two Brothers[244] Endoscopy, anatomical, chemical and textile analysis, radiology 1992 Natsefamun Endoscopy, Radiology 1975 Mummy 1770 Radiology, CAT scans, MRI, histology, electron microscopy, carbon dating, serology, DNA studies, fingerprint, dental exam and facial reconstruction, endoscopy, samples taken. 2001 Asru Endoscopy, Radiology
Sir Marc Armand Ruffer, London[245]	1909-1913 Several mummies and mummy parts Paleopathology pioneer
National Museum of Leiden[246]	1960 Radiology 1970 CAT scans 1997 New CAT scans to all mummies 133 mummies, the oldest from the XXth Dynasty, most of them from the Third Intermediate period to Greco-Roman period
Aidan Cockburn, Detroit Institute of Arts	1972-1973 Mummy PUM I e PUM II Autopsies
Musée de l'Homme de Paris[247]	1975 Ramesses II Radiology, specialized lab exam
Toronto, Royal Ontario Museum, Canada	1974 Nakht-ROM I Autopsy, radiology
James E. Harris, University of Michigan, Ann Arbor, USA[248]	1980 Makare, Nodjme Macroscopical exam, radiology Seti I Siptah Ramesses II Macroscopical exam, radiology

Authors	Date and tests conducted
Department of radiology, University Hospital, Pennsylvannia[249]	1980 Djedhapi Macroscopical exam, radiology Hapimen Macroscopical exam, radiology PUM II (Pennsylvania University Museum II) Autopsy
Niagara Falls Egyptian Museum Collection, USA[250]	1980's 9 Mummies Study of mummy labels, radiology, endoscopy, tissue samples taken
Uppsala University, Sweden[251]	1985 Skin and bone samples taken from 23 mummies
Lakehead University, Ontario, Canada, project from the Dakhla Oasis in the western Egyptian desert	Since 1986 bone and tissue analysis Since 1996 X-ray analysis More than 3000 graves, 300 analyzed until 2006
The Oriental Institute Museum, University, Chicago, USA	1991 Meresamun MRI
	1991 PetOsiris CAT scans, MRI, radiology
Archaeological Collection from Belgrade Faculty of Philosophy[252]	Since May 1993 Mummy, adult Samples were chemically analyzed
Brigham Young University, USA	1993-94 DNA studies, 6 mummies from the Old Kingdom
Cracow Archaeological Museum, Poland[253]	1995 Isitirikhetes, Ptolemaic period, IV to I centuries BC CAT scans, physical-chemical exam, serology, histology
Egyptian Museum Cairo	1990's DNA studies 27 royal mummies from the New Kingdom[254] Seven had successful results

[243] KNH Centre , Manchester:
http://www.ls.manchester.ac.uk/egyptology/
[244] http://www.archive.org/details/tomboftwobrother00murr
[245] Ruffer, 1910 (várias páginas; praticamente toda esta obra é uma compilação de exames a múmias egípcias servindo portanto de referência neste tipo de estudo e indicada em todas as bibliografias correspondentes à área da bio medicina em Egyptlogia).
[246] Published in Maarten J. Raven, Wybren K. Taconis, R. W. R. J. Dekker, *Egyptian Mummies: Radiological Atlas of the Collections in the National Museum of Antiquities at Leiden, Papers on Archaeology of the Leiden Museum of Antiquities.*
[247] Published in Balout, L., *La momie de Ramsès II au Musée de l'Homme, Le Courrier du CNRS*, 28, 1978: 38-42 and in Balout, Lionel, *La Momie de Ramsès II, Contribution scientifique à l'Égyptologie sous la direction de Lionel Balout et C. Roubet, avec la participation de Christiane Desroches-Noblecourt*, Éditions Recherche sur les Civilisations, Paris, 1985.
[248] Fleming, Fishman, O'Connor, Silverman, 1980:60, 62, 84, 85.

[249] Fleming, Fishman, O'Connor, Silverman, 1980:82, 83, 87-89.
[250] Collection started in the 1850's, when Sydney Barnett, son of the Museum founder, Thomas Barnett, went to Egypt to purchase some antiquities: http://www.egyptianMuseumm.com/mummies.html; articles published: http://www.egyptianMuseumm.com/article_index.html
[251] Pääbo, 1985: 411-417; Pääbo, 1985: 644-645; Pääbo, 1986: 441-446.
[252] http://dekart.f.bg.ac.yu/~bandjelk/bemum/index.html
[253] Polish Academy of Arts and Sciences, 2001; The Gods of Ancient Egypt, 2003.
[254] Photos in digital version of *Catalogue General Antiquités Egyptiennes du Musée du Caire: The Royal Mummies* in http://www.lib.uchicago.edu/cgi-bin/eos/eos_title.pl?callnum=DT57.C2_vol59

Authors	Date and tests conducted
Wilfred Griggs, Scott Woodward, Rosicrucian Egyptian Museum, San Jose, California, USA Stanford University, California, USA, Rosicrucian Egyptian Museum, San Jose, California, USA	August 1995 6 mummies: Nesimin, Tuhere, Usermontu, Irtieru, unknown woman and child (4 to 6 years old) DNA studies, tissue analysis May 2005 Cherit CAT scans April 2007 Mummy, female, Rosicrucian Egyptian Museum, California, 4-5 years of age CAT scan for tri-dimensional reconstruction
Egyptian and Rosacruz Museum, Curitiba, Brasil	1997 (since) "Thotmea" Unwrapped in 1888, exhibited, CAT scans, Radiology
Royal Ontario Museum, Canada	1995/96 DjedMaatiuesankh CAT scans, radiology
Emory University, Atlanta, USA	March 2000 Ramesses I Radiology, CAT scans for tri-dimensional reconstruction
Fine Arts Museum, San Francisco, USA	May 13, 2000 Mummy, adult CAT scans
Akhmim Mummy Studies Consortium[255] Harrisburg, Pennsylvania, USA Berkshire Museum, USA, Jonathan Elias Akhmim Mummy Studies Consortium	August 2001 to June 2006 13 mummies from several locations CAT scans June 2007 Pahat CAT for tri-dimensional reconstruction
New Wilmington College, Reading Public Museum, Pennsylvania, USA	November 2003 Pesed CAT scans, radiology
Djehuti, Heri, Tombs, Dra Abu el-Naga, Luxor by Salima Ikram	2004 2 mummies and 4 human heads
Nicholson Museum Egyptian Mummy Project, University of Sydney, Australia	2004 Padiachaikhet CAT scans and tests find tuberculosis and hepatitis B
Centre de Researchs Renato Archer (CenPRA), Ministério da Ciencia e Tecnologia (MCT), Campinas (SP), Brasil[256]	August 2004 Lecture about the technical aspects of virtual reconstruction of mummies by CAT scans, graphic computation and prototyping for study and identification. Presentation about the collection from the National Museum in Rio de January and ongoing project, with CenPRA and Instituto Nacional de Tecnologia (INT), showing preliminary results.
Madeeha Khattab's team Dean from the School of Medicine of University Cairo, with specialists from Italy and Switzerland.	2005 Tutankhamun CAT scans National Geographic Society and Siemens Medical Solutions donated the equipment.

Authors	Date and tests conducted
Royal Museums of Scotland, Edinburgh	March 2005 Nubian queen and son Infrared, tri-dimensional reconstruction
British Museum, London	May 2005 Shepenmehit (f), a boy, a young male, Padiamenet (m), Tjaiasetimu (f), Irethoreru (m) CAT scans
University de Munich Ludwig-Maximilians	October 2006 91 Egyptian mummies, 70 Nubian mummies DNA samples from bones
Carnegie Museum of Natural History, University of Pittsburgh School of Medicine, USA	May 2007 Mummy from the Ptolemaic period, between 3 and 5 years old. It was discovered in 1912 by Henri Naville in a cemetery from Abydos. It was in a tomb with seven other adults and four children. It is the only one in good condition to be exhibited, so it was sent to the Carnegie Museum. In 1986, doctors from the Forbes Metropolitan Health Centre, Wilkinsburg took some X-rays.
Egyptian Museum Cairo, Applied Biosystems[257]	June 2007 Hatshepsut CAT scans, DNA studies

An important detail to mention is that foreign politics (the Big Depression of 1929, the two World Wars and post-war reconstruction) have delayed the progress of biomedical science in Egyptology, between the 1930's and the 1970's from the 20th century. But the main purpose for the facial tri-dimensional reconstruction of mummies undertaken on several occasions over last few years is that it is important both anthropologically, for medicine and also for forensic purposes. The aim of these studies is to use a multi-detector examination CAT scans for facial tri-dimensional reconstruction and report the results from a multidisciplinary team of radiologists, anthropologists and forensic scientists in the reconstitution/reconstruction of a probable physiognomy of an ancient Egyptian.

---

[255] http://amscresearch.com/_wsn/page2.html
[256] http://www.int.gov.br/Novo/Menus/mumia.html; Jornal da Ciência September, 30, 2002
http://www.jornaldaciencia.org.br/Detalhe.jsp?id=5131

[257] Zahi Hawass describes all the process from the discovery of the tomb (KV60) by Carter in 1903 until 1989 when Zahi Hawass visited the location and decides to bring the mummy to Cairo Egyptian Museum. The tests started with the canopic vases containing residues from the organs of Hatshepsut and only after they radiographed the box containing the liver, stomach and tooth (2005-2006); the tooth was a perfect match to the empty alveolar hole from the obese mummy at KV60 and, in July 2007 DNA tests were done to this mummy identifying it as Hatshepsut. CAT scans were done and the very preliminary results indicate that there is a probability of her having diabetes, she had also bad dentition and might have had cancer. This laboratory was built in the basement of the Cairo Museum, but, Zahi Hawass intends also to build another lab in the National Research Centre in Dokki, Cairo. In an interview given in April 2007, Zahi Hawass referred the following data regarding Hatshepsut: the one that was considered the 'nanny' because she was middle-aged (about 50 with skin layers of fat) was brought by Howard Carter to the Cairo Museum in 1907. A curious fact is that, all these mummies from the XVIIIth Dynasty did not have an eviscerated brain, according to Zahi Hawass:
http://www.guardians.net/hawass/hatshepsut/search_for_hatshepsut.htm

An original research has been done by Jacqueline Finch, on mummy prosthetics for arm and foot. The prosthetic might have been used to create personal symmetry.[258]

---

[258] Finch, 2005: 43. The foot is part of Finch's PhD project at Manchester's KNH Centre.

Chapter 2

Heka – ⌐⏀⌐ "the art of the magical written word"

Sir James George Frazer defines magic as "the manipulation of supernatural beings by a human who expects that the correct sequence of words or actions will automatically bring about the desired result. "[259]

"Ten measures of witchcraft descended to the world; nine were taken by Egypt. "[260]

Herman Te Velde describes magic as: "The distinction between the magical and the religious is one of definition. The word magic is often used simply to label actions, sayings, and ideas that do not seem reasonable from a Western positivist or Christian point of view. "[261]

Criterion, category or concept, the word *magic* is used to describe the activities of the doctor-magician as action. According to Panagiotis Kousoulis[262] "to understand *heka*, magic, is essential for our knowledge of Egyptian cosmos ". *heka* was a natural force, but could also be represented as god in human form".[263] Magic would eventually keep the body in harmony with the cosmos so that this would be a receptacle, capable of incorporating vital forces. The importance of magic is its gift to allow humans to fight material and spiritual dangers by faith.

In the *Rollin Papyrus*, dating unknown, describing a magical practice it is said: "it happened because the writings were conceived to spell, banish and confuse"[264]
In the *Lee Papyrus,* dealing also with magical causes it is said: "…I have not given any writing to no one (…) give me a piece of writing so I can have power and authority"[265]

The magician Djedjemankh is referred to in the *Westcar Papyrus*, in the tales of Khufu, in a story about Khufu's father, Senefru. In this, Dedi said his "saying of magic and separated the lake waters" to search and collect a lost pendant, fallen from a barge.[266]
The ancient Egyptians saw the universe as if it had no movement at all; static. They thought, we think, after looking at their writings and art depictions, that the cosmic order would have been created once and ... that is all. This order would be disturbed many times by the

forces of chaos promptly dominated, but never annihilated. This coherence in thought, in such a linear way in opposition to the universe, was placed in the daily earthly life. Maybe the geographic conditions, different today but at that time they were uniform across the country, promoted a sense of continuity, for example, the annual flood which happened at a precise date in the calendar. The abundance and pleasure represented in tomb scenes and writings of ancient Egypt reflected this continuity, eternal, of the life they had on Earth.

In ancient Egypt the word used for magic was *heka*; deriving from the Greek *mageia*.[267]

This word is used in ancient Egypt since The Pyramid Texts from the Old Kingdom until the Coptic period, where it becomes *hik*.[268] The word *hik* from Coptic origin during the first years of Christianity was the equivalent to *mageia* (Greek) and *magia* (Latin); *heka*[269] had no negative or illegal connotations. Although magic was somehow 'condemned' in Antiquity it was practised by those who preferred to see it as a means of protection or defence from another entity.[270] Magic became the irrational precursor of science.[271] The Arabic word *baraka*,[272] a blessing, is also linked with *heka*.

It was *heka* who revived the deceased in the Afterlife and allowed both the *ka* and the *ba* from the deceased to work in the name of him/her in the afterlife. The power of magic was associated to the power of word, written or spoken, as the word represented the essence of it, and therefore acted upon it. The oral rituals had a great reputation for power; reciting, as it is seen in the descriptions from the ritual of the opening of the mouth of the deceased's mummy, was believed to confer life to him/her.

In Chapter 23 from The Book of the Dead there is a formula to open the mouth of the deceased in the

---

[259] Pinch, 1994: 12.
[260] Talmud (Rabbinic writings from Orthodox Jews), Kiddushin 49b (literally the sanctification). It is the first part of the Jewish matrimony that creates the legal bond without the mutual bond.
[261] Quoted by Meyer, Smith, 1994: 13.
[262] Panagiotis Kousoulis, specialist on magic and medicine in ancient Egypt;
http://www.rhodes.aegean.gr/tms/DEP_personal_pages/Kousoulis/CVKousoulis%200706.pdf
[263] Meyer, Smith, 1994: 15; Kousoulis, 2001.
[264] Goedicke, 1963: 72.
[265] Goedicke, 1963: 78.
[266] Lichtheim, 1973, 2006: 216-217.

[267] Who practice the *mageia*: the *magos*. The word *magoi* appears four times in the second chapter of the Greek Gospel of Matthew, the Vulgata translates the word as *magi*. In English translations the word appears as 'wise men', *magos* being an import from the Persian, according to Porphyry, and this word means interpreter or divine adorator. The wise men at Jesus' birth would probably have been *magos* in the magical sense.
[268] Meyer, Smith, 1994: 14.
[269] Ritner, 1993: 15.
[270] Meyer, Smith, 1994: 2.
[271] Meyer, Smith, 1994: 3.
[272] Pinch, 1994:12. *Berakhah, berakhah* or *bracha*, in Hebrew: ברכה; plural ברכות, *berakhot* is a blessing, usually recited in a specific moment. *Baraka* or *Barakah* in Arabic, بركة , is a word referring to the divine presence, charisma, wisdom or blessing transmitted from a tutor to a disciple. Both Hebrew and Arabic are derived from Aramaic so we can conclude that these words reflect the same concept.

kingdom of the deceased which illustrates power of the word pronounced out loud:

" My mouth is released by Ptah;
the bonds of my mouth are caused to be unfettered by the god of my city.
Thoth comes fully equipped with his words of power,
and has released for me the items belonging to Seth, the bonds of my mouth,
My hands are moved by Atum, he puts them forward as the guard of my mouth.
My mouth is opened, my mouth is parted by Ptah with that tool of iron,
with which he has opened the mouth of the gods.
I am Sekhmet Wadjyt,
I sit beside the great starboard in the sky,
I am Sahyt amidst the powers of Iunu.
As for any words of power, any speech uttered against me,
May the gods stand against them, the assembled Ennead and its Enneads. "[273]

In this Chapter of the Book of the Dead there is an attempt to syncretically associate several divinities from different cosmogonies in a characteristic so Egyptian as to never obliterate any divinity or a group of divinities, explaining their existence in the hierarchy as new divinities appear. Ptah (from the Memphite cosmogony) and Thoth (from the hermopolitan cosmogony) come together to help the deceased as well as all the Eneade (we suppose the Heliopolis one, from the text).

The use of the two fingers (index and second finger from the right hand) restored the use of the senses in the deceased.[274]

The *akh* was the transfigured spirit of the deceased[275] which, after passing the Judgement on the weighting of the heart, attested the truth of his/her affirmations regarding his/her earthly life, although later, in the Greco-Roman period, *akh* usually designates a demon.[276]

A stela from the 4th century BC, at the temple of Khonsu at Karnak (C 284, Louvre), describes an event which occurred in the reign of Ramesses II, in which a princess, Bentresh, sister of the Hittite wife of the king, was very sick in her kingdom. A scribe did the diagnosis and Ramesses II sends a Khonsu statue to treat the princess. The spirit gave in before the offerings of the princess' father so that it would abandon her.[277]

Funerary magic had the aim of helping the deceased to deal with demons to be found in his/her way. In popular magic there were complex beings, hybrids, pantheistic divinities that combine qualities and attributes from different gods. Several qualities of strong animals in only one divinity, as the Big Eater present at the Final Judgement of the deceased with a hippopotamus head, a lion body and crocodile paws.

She represented the imminent punishment just in case the deceased's heart revealed sins practised against Maat therefore, lies against the gods. The rituals such as The Opening of the Mouth, as well as the ears, eyes, and nose were used so that the deceased could recover his/her senses in the afterlife. The name of this ritual comes from texts of funerary liturgy where it was recited over the mummy, while the mouth was opened so that the deceased had voice in the underworld.[278] It helped to develop the quality of *maat-kheru* or justified. This stage was only reached by the ones who passed the final judgement of the actions they performed in life. By the negative, the deceased stated everything bad he/she did not commit and that was confirmed comparing the weight of his/her heart on the scales against a Maat feather. Anubis, the son of Osiris and Nephtys, controlled the event. Thoth took notes of everything happening, as a court officer would do. Whoever attained the condition of 'justified' became *akh*, a transfigured spirit and could join the gods.

A spell could be made to conjure spirits from the underworld based on sympathetic magic, performing alterations in living or inanimate objects through a model. Speechless, blindness, paralysis, physical impairment or even death could be caused. Statuettes of human figures were used to cast a spell in the intended person imitating him/her with real hair and papyrus in the back (the examples are from the Greco-Roman period). The technique consisted in mixing the person's own hair[279] with a deceased person's hair; (example at the British Museum), statuette of a woman with hands tied at the back and nails in her body (another example at the Louvre). These statuettes were buried near the tomb of a young woman or someone that have died of a violent death, reflecting a relationship of love/hate.

The ideas about *heka* could have been Egyptian but the words are almost totally Greek. The Papyri that survived until today do not make a distinction between magic and medicine. They group sections of treatment according to the affected body part or complaint but as a psychosomatic practice; preventive medicine was essentially magic. Ancient Egyptians used magic to deal with health problems or cast away foreign enemies. Magic solved crises and was also prophylactic. The causes of misfortune could be several; magic applies the cure defending the human against the will of the gods.

The mouth has an essential role in magic; the pronounced knowing, the reciting of a spell[280] or the ingestion of

---

[273] University College London:
http://www.digitalegypt.ucl.ac.uk/literature/religious/bd23.html
[274] Germond, 2005: 97.
[275] Pinch, 1994: 147.
[276] Pinch, 1994: 45.
[277] Lichtheim, 1997: 134-136.

[278] With a *pesechkef*, further explained in this work.
[279] Pinch, 1994: 160.
[280] Pinch, 1994: 154.

ingredients consolidated magic;[281] to lick a spell, to spit or to vomit upon a name, someone or a written spell, had magical characteristics.

To swallow, as a magical act, is very well documented: it is a synonym of wisdom, physically and metaphorically, and it can mean both the destruction of what is ingested or its infusion of magic or both.[282]

It was a custom practice to write letters to relatives of the deceased requiring intercession so that a spell was effective.[283] This ancient Egyptian practice of letters with complaints presented to the gods and deceased relatives, threatening the divinities to force them to agree, lasts until the Coptic period.[284]

The hands (*djrt*, hand), were used as representations of genitals and were referred to as "Lady of the Vulva" or "Hand of Atum"[285] in connection to the myth where he used his hand to masturbate himself and create his children Shu, the air and Tefnut, the humidity in the creation of the Cosmos.

The feet, (*rd*, foot), were also used in the ritual of stomping the enemy through figures representing the feet drawn in the interior soles of sandals[286] and on the exterior face of sarcophagus' feet.

To step on, to beat and to burn a wax figure was a common practice.[287]

Throwing sticks as it is depicted in the tomb of Nakht, was used to cast away birds[288] and in a ritual way, also to cast away demons, and all sorts of amulets were used to protect the deceased on his/her journey to the afterlife, wrapped within the linen bandages of the mummy.

Other ritual acts such as walking around an object, house[289] or shrine, were connected by the word magic, and it was the responsibility of the magician to persuade the gods of this connection between the cosmic and the real world, trying to convince them to come in his aid. But magic was not always beneficial; there was also the dark side[290]... spells were made against enemies of the king ... lists with their names that were crushed, burnt, pierced, buried and boiled in urine...

The power of images and words was increased when carved in stone for eternity; thus an event such as the death of Osiris was too awful to be shown; and to portray

any triumph, even temporary, from the forces of evil, might give them strength to act in the real world. Osiris was the most vulnerable god and because of that, the most explored in magic. The ancient Egyptians considered magic as a cosmic force of neutral moral. *heka* or the creator[291] was also *ba*, manifestation of the solar god represented in human form with a magical wand in the shape of a snake.

In the Coffin Spells n.261 there is a reference to the solar role of magic in creation and as *heka* it can also be the creator. Between the perception that takes place in the heart (or spirit of the deceased), and the annunciation that comes by word, this spell n.261 identifies that ability in the deceased and gives him/her power to act.[292]

All the performers of magic had to know which amulets to use, what blessings to give, what offerings to give and to whom, what prayers to read and when, the right locations to give devotion to, such as to prevent bad luck when travelling and to be aware of the beneficial and the nefast days in the calendar.[293] In the British Museum there is *Papyrus* 10184, from Saqqara, from the end of the XIXth Dynasty, c. 1225 BC, a calendar with advice to live day-by-day as the Egyptian calendar classified the days in those two categories.

Another example is the one from *Papyrus Sallier* IV also in the British Museum where days are listed accordingly; what to do and what not to do on particular days. Certain rites of purification, abstinence and cleanliness were asked from performers of magic as well as the purification of spaces, using magical wands many times so that a magic would be more effective. In the *Ebers Papyrus* the contents were both medical and magical simultaneously; among the medical procedures we find also spells. There was no distinction between science and religion; between magic and reason.

Many magical/religious treatments tried to fight diseases caused in humans by magic of the gods, bad spirits, all types of *whdw*, a pain, according to Nunn;[294] (a putrefact substance[295] noxious, pus,[296] toxin[297] or even more than that,[298] one that the body receives as an invader, a pathological entity[299] causing evil to the body and spirit).

According to José das Candeias Sales magic could be divided in three different types: religious, popular and profane.[300]

---

[281] Pinch, 1994: 136.
[282] DuQuesne, 2006: 23.
[283] Ritner, 1993: 180-183; Petrie Museum of Egyptian Archaeology at University College London http://www.petrie.ucl.ac.uk/index2.html
[284] Meyer, Smith, 1994: 185.
[285] Noegel, 2004.
[286] Pinch, 1994: 115.
[287] Meyer, Smith, 1994: 185-186.
[288] Fleming, Fishman, O'Connor, Silverman, 1980:78-79.
[289] Pinch, 1994: 143.
[290] Pinch, 1994:156.

[291] Allen, 1997: 17.
[292] Allen, 1997: 17.
[293] Pinch, 1994: 158.
[294] Nunn, 1996: 61.
[295] Nunn, 1996: 62.
[296] Nunn, 1996: 76, 166.
[297] Nunn, 1996: 158.
[298] Nunn, 1996: 85.
[299] Nunn, 1996: 105.
[300] Sales, 1999: 81.

The religious type, with medicinal character, was found in practices from the temples and rituals, as The Pyramid Texts, The Coffin Spells, and The Book of the Dead, *prt m hru*, The Book of Going Forth by the Day, the mummies' linen inscriptions and the tomb walls' inscriptions as well as the writings on the sarcophagi.

The popular magic, practised at home, linked to personal beliefs using and abusing amulets, and the profane, as shown in the tales from the *Westcar Papyrus*, in which the aim was to improve the magical strength of the performer, the magician, focused on word.

In Greek, Coptic and Demotic texts 450 substances are mentioned as pharmacologically active in spells, formulas and requests.[301]

2.1. The performance: priests, exorcists, doctors-magicians

In a society where writing and reading were reserved for scribes, priests, kings and notable people, they would have seemed to be magicians by the rest of the population, as they mastered the word and all written word had power.

The Egyptian concept of power concealed in the pronounced word could be used both with good or bad intentions, a note: Egyptologists distance themselves from the study of the occult, but the study of magic in ancient Egypt portrays their society and this would be incomplete without the element of magic.

The professionals of *heka* (magic) were also called physicians (doctors), as *heka* was associated with medicine and with the divine world in general.

The performers of *heka* are the *hekau* and they can be priests; especially lector-priests,[302] although there were other terms linked to these performers of magical acts, funerary *sem* priests, and Sekhmet priests.[303]

All those born with physical deformities or different visible abnormalities such as dwarfs, *nemu*, were considered as possessing magical qualities. The lector-priests, intimately associated with religious ceremonies, magic and reading/casting of spells, were the ones speaking the magical words during ceremonies. Some doctors, *sunu*, became known as lector-priests also. Some examples are: Mereruka, a doctor, son-in-law and vizier of Teti in the VIth Dynasty, and Hui, from the kingdom of Amenhotep III, who gave him the title of "Chief of the Secrets of the Palace", he was also vice-king of Nubia under the kingdom of Tutankhamun, and he is represented in the temple of Seti I at Abydos, he was

considered a wise man and legends say that he lived until 110 years of age.

Doctors had assistants,[304] nurses, mid-wives, physical therapists and bandagists wrapping the patients' wounds;[305] these were specialists and as Herodotus said[306] (II, 84), "the art of medicine divided between those: each doctor is dedicated to one disease, and no more. All the places have plenty of doctors; some doctors are for the eyes, others for the head, others for the teeth and others for the belly and others for internal disorders". Herodotus was too distant in specifying these doctors' specializations; there were general performers; maybe he did not mention this because it was too obvious! Ophthalmology was practised in abundance as blindness and eye diseases were common in ancient Egypt and trachoma, for example, was as prevalent then as it is today. Sete oculists (ophtalmologists) were identified in ancient Egypt.

There were also specialists of internal medicine, as we call it today, gynaecologists and some other speciality as the "guardian of the anus"; probably the proctologist.

There were also doctors for the cemeteries and in the Middle Kingdom a doctor for the troops is also registered,[307] in the New Kingdom there was the title of Chief of The House of Life[308] which seems to be an administrative function like a minister of health.

There were also dentists and manufacturers of false teeth, doctors for the boats that sailed out of Ancient Egypt and even miners had their own doctors.

The priest Hor, c. 200 BC, is an example of someone who dedicated his life serving Thoth, after having received divine visions.

The priest-doctor-magician is also the pharmacist, as he is the one preparing the ingredients to use, and his material compositions were accompanied by spiritual concepts according to what was considered to improve the efficacy of the medicine.[309] All must have begun with Thoth, who was called the first doctor, and the first surgeon; s*unu*.[310] Some magicians had tattoos of Osiris on their shoulders, to identify themselves with Thoth.

The day and the hour for the ritual/spell were chosen according to the calendar of beneficial days. The magician had to prepare himself by purifying his body;

[301] University of Arkansas, Fayetteville, Arkansas, USA; http://www.uark.edu/campus-resources/dlevine/Magika5.html
[302] Meyer, Smith, 1994: 15.
[303] Pinch, 1994: 54.
[304] Pinch, 1994: 140.
[305] Nunn, 1996: 32-33.
[306] Herodotus, 2003: 127.
[307] Doctors list (table) further shown in this work: *Sunu sa*, troops' doctor, Akemu, Middle Kingdom.
[308] Jonckheere, 1958: 42.
[309] Nunn, 1996: 132.
[310] Sullivan, 1996: 467, Grapow uses *sinu* based on the Coptic concept *met* for doctor, preceded of the prefix *caein*; *metcaein* or *metchini* that originated the word medicine. The prefix is added to the name, *metceni*. There is no doubt about the use of *sinu* for doctor as demonstrated by Jonckheere, 1958, and Nunn, 1996:115.

washing his mouth and ears with natron. The magician had to abstain himself from having sex for three or seven days depending on the ritual. According to Geraldine Pinch[311] in the *Book of the Heavenly Cow*, a priest performing magic painted the image of Maat on his tongue so that his words came out truthfully. The magician also transferred the hurtful effects of poison or spirit to an object that was then crushed, buried or driven by the Nile waters.

The performer expresses the will of the supernatural powers by personifying them, according to Borghouts, in *Ancient Egyptian Magical Texts*.[312]

Medical diagnostic

In ancient Egypt all diagnostics began by: "you should say about him (the patient) .... "[313]

Then, after examining the patient, the doctor has three options, and will say one of the following about the state of the patient: "a disease I can (will) treat" – used in situations of guaranteed cure; "a disease I will try to treat" – used for difficult cases but not impossible ones. The doctor will try to treat it but the result is unforeseen; "a disease not treatable" – in these cases the situation cannot be resolved by the doctor because he thinks it is incurable. Therefore magic will be used. The doctor cast away the spirit; it was impossible to distinguish in which time he was the physician and which time he was the magician or priest.

According to the *Edwin Smith Papyrus*, case 1, "all the *uab* priest of Sekhmet, all the *sa* (Serket), that puts his hands or fingers over a head, back of the head, hands, the place of the heart, the legs, it is to the heart-*haty* that the exam is made to, as the channels/vessels *metu* of the man are all over his body and it is the (heart-*haty*), that speaks to the channels/vessels *metu* that belong to each part of the body." [314]

There were several categories of doctors for the public and for the royals, in records from ancient Egypt:

---

[311] Pinch, 1994: 77-78
[312] Also quoted in Meyer, Smith, 1994: 17.
[313] Nunn, 1996: 114; Sipos, Gyory, Hagymási, Onderjka, Blázovics, 2004: 214.

[314] Bardinet, 1995: 85 (*Ebers Papyrus* 854a); Badiola: 48; 494 (*Edwin Smith Papyrus*); Nunn, 1996:113.

Doctors' name [315]	*Sunu* plus	Title	Some known names[316] and period
Imit re sunu		Chief of female doctors	Peseshet,[317] Old Kingdom (OK)
Kherep sunu	*Pera* (from the palace)	Administractr of doctors	
Heri sunu	*N nesu* (from the king)	The one with authority over the doctors	
Imir sunu	*Neb taui* (of the two lands)	Supervisor of doctors	*Sunu n neb taui*
Sehedj sunu	*N per hemet nesu* (of the queen)	Inspector of doctors	*Sehedj sunu* Irenakhti III, OK Hunennefer I, OK Hunennefer II, OK Niankhknum, OK Nesemnau (several titles),[318] OK Kaudja I, OK
Uer sunu	*Iret pera* (Chief of the oculists of the palace) *Uer sunu mehu chema* (Chief of doctors of Lower and Upper Egypt) *Uer sunu m ast Maat* (Chief of doctors of the place of Truth – Necropolis) *Uer sunu n hat ankh* (Chief dos doctors da House de Life)	Chief of doctors	Imeni Amenhotep, New Kingdom (NK) Ankh I, OK Antiemhat, Middle Kingdom (MK) Udjahoresnet, LP Paieftauherauineit, Later period(LP) Penthu, NK Psemtekseneb (several titles),[319] LP Niankh-sekhmet, (several titles)[320] Kingdom Ancient Nespamedu, LP Nedjemu, MK Kamose NK Renefseneb MK Hi, NK *Uer sunu* Sankh-khnum, MK

---

[315] Adapted from Nunn, 1996: 117-118.
[316] Jonckheere, 1958: 18-77.
[317] Peseshet had another title: *imit-re hem (ut) -ka*, Chief of the priestesses of the soul, who dealt with private funerals: Ghalioungui, 1975: 113.
[318] Jonckheere, 1958: 56.
[319] Jonckheere, 1958: 40. His statue was originally at Sais.
[320] Jonchkeere, 1958: 49.

			Seni, MK
		.	Gua, MK (irhand de Seni)
			Uer sunu pera
			Heremakhbit, LP
			Uer sunu iret pera
			Uahduau, OK
			Uer sunu mehu chema
			Paanmeniu, LP
			Uer sunu m ast Maat
			Puer, NK
			Uer sunu n hat ankh
			Menna, NK
Sunu	*Iret* (oculist, ophthalmologist) *Hat iret* (doctor of womb and eyes) *Sunu n per imn* (medical do temple de Amun) *Sunu n per hemet nesut* (medical da House da Esposa do King)	Medical	Ankh III
			Impi, MK
			Paraemheb
			Mehu
			Neferher, NK
			Neferherenptah, OK
			Nekht, MK
			Nekht-hedj-es
			Rediemptah
			Hui, LP
			Hormes
			Hetep-akhty
			Kaimin, NK
			Kaudja II
			Thuthu, NK
			Netherhetep
			Sunu pera
			Ipi II, OK
			Irenakhti I, OK
			Irenakhti II (several titles),[321] OK
			Ptahotep, OK
			Mer-Pepi, OK
			Medunefer, OK
			Niankhknum, OK
			Kuy, OK
			Sunu iret
			Uai I, OK
			Sunu hat iret
			Uai II, LP
			Neferthes, OK
			Sunu n per imn
			Pahaiatu
			Sunu n per hemet nesut
			Ra, NK
			Kai, NK
ChemShu sunu pera			Ankh II
			Bebi, OK
			Neferi, MK
			Djau I, OK
			Djau II, OK
Sunu gereget[322]		Doctor of the colony	Methen, OK
Sunu sa[323]		Doctor of the troops	Akemu, MK
Iri ibeh		Dentist	Menkaureankh Nefer-iret-es, OK
Seche sunu n nisut		Scribe and doctor of the king	NebAmun, NK

[321] Jonckheere, 1958: 25.
[322] Ebeid, 1999: 330; Jonckheere, 1958: 46.
[323] Jonckheere, 1958: 29, 103.

Around c. 2000 BC, doctors had a salary, whether they were employed by the temple or by the army to accompany military campaigns and treat the men. They did not charge for their services, but they charged for the prescriptions they made.[324] Diodorus Siculus speaks about the medical profession as being paid by the State, saying that, if the doctor follows the law and does not heal the patient his guilt is pardoned but, if, by the contrary he does not follow the law and the patient dies, there will be a trial, and the doctor can be sentenced to death.[325] Therefore, there was no room for independent practices and all doctors followed what was written in the sacred books for a long time.

The work was an occupation with few hygiene patterns defined at that time, and it was a dangerous profession for health. From fractures due to trauma; accidents carrying weights, to eye infections and skin eruptions due to the desert winds blowing, limited personal hygiene habits during work times, small riots between workers, food poisoning and teeth and mouth decay, heat and insect plagues, all were contributions for several incapacities.
While the pyramids were being built, support medical services were assured; Methen was the *sunu gereget* or colony doctor assigned for the work field.[326] The workers had medical insurance; an interesting text describes a worker being attacked in one eye while at work and being discharged for his incapacity, he was then readmitted after allegedly stating it was a work accident and he demanded from the temple his payment and the cost of his treatment. There was no age limit for retirement except in the case of physical incapacity.[327]

Anastasi Papyrus IV shows that workers had the right to a pension fund in case of incapacity.[328] Casualties due to disease were allowed. An ostracon from the year 40 of Ramesses II (XIX Dynasty, 1240 BC) has a list of forty names with absentees at work, the most frequent cause being disease.[329]

The strike is described in the *Turin Papyrus* 2044[330] where more information is given; neither sick nor wounded workers can lift stones.[331] The work schedule was four hours in the morning and four hours in the afternoon, with a meal and 'siesta' in the middle of the two periods of work to avoid sunburn. There were medical structures to support the neighbourhoods.[332]

Peseshet

Peseshet, from the Vth or VIth Dynasty (c. 2350-2320 BC), the first female doctor, *imi-rá sunut*,[333] *imit-rá sunu*,[334] supervisor of the funerary priestesses, allows us to conclude that there were already female doctors in the Old Kingdom. There were fewer women in this profession maybe because of the restriction on learning to read and write.
Menstruation could also be an impediment to the exercise of this profession as menstruating women were considered impure. Also because women who had died were sometimes considered powerful demons, they were feared, especially the magic from foreigners (Nubian) but even so, some doctors would possibly have female assistants.
Having Sekhmet as 'godmother', all doctors succeeded in their careers by merit and this should have happened also with Peseshet. Could she have been an experimental gynaecologist interrupting pregnancies, treating difficult and painful menstruations and diagnosing cancers in the uterus; being an obstetrician? Why are there no more records of women in this profession?[335]

Excavations at the tomb of AkhetHotep in Giza revealed a monument dedicated to Peseshet, identified as the supervisor of female doctors; not simple midwives.[336] In *Excavations at Giza I*, 1929-1930, Selim Hassan published the stela of Peseshet, discovered in this tomb from the Old Kingdom. In fact, the word supervisor exists in the female. And *sunu*, doctor, is written with the *t* characteristic of the female.[337]

Imhotep

Doctor known as having existed under the reign of king Djoser, IIIth Dynasty, c. 2700-2625 BC, also an architect, he was an educated man and he was known also as the builder of the first step pyramid of Saqqara. He was worshipped later as the god of medicine, the prototype of Asclepius, as Thoth was the prototype of Hermes and Mercury and the first of doctors. We know little about Imhotep and his medical knowledge but his apotheosis is meaningful enough to say that he was the first recorded man in ancient Egyptian medicine.

As a doctor, Imhotep is thought to be the author, according to the *Edwin Smith Papyrus*, of ninety anatomical writings and the description of 48 wounds. He founded a school of medicine in Memphis; he diagnosed and treated about two hundred diseases, fifteen diseases of the abdomen, eleven of the bladder, ten of the rectum, 29 of the eyes, and eighteen of the skin, hair, tongue, tuberculosis, bladder stones, appendicitis and arthritis. He also practised surgery[338] and was a dentist, he knew the

[324] Justin, 2003: 276.
[325] Nunn, 1996: 121.
[326] Jonckheere, 1958: 102.
[327] Sameh, 2000.
[328] Lisboa, 1978: 284.
[329] Ebeid, 1999: 328.
[330] Papyrus from Deir el-Medina at the Egyptian Museum of Turin.
[331] Ebeid, 1999: 333.
[332] Ebeid, 1999: 329-330; Sameh, 2000; Papyrus referenced in the Deir el-Medina Database, *A Survey of the New Kingdom Non-literary Texts from Deir el-Medina*, Leiden University; http://www.wepwawet.nl/dmd/guide.htm, published in Botti, G. e T.E. Peet, *Il giornale della necropoli di Tebe* (I papiri ieratici del Museo di Torino), Turin, 1928.

[333] Nunn, 1996: 124.
[334] Jonckheere, 1958: 41.
[335] Ghalioungui, 1975: 163.
[336] Ebeid, 1999: 74-75.
[337] Cuenca-Estrella, 2004: 59.
[338] From the Greek *kheirourgía* that means work by hand.

position and function of the organs and he knew about the circulation of blood in the human organism. His tomb at Saqqara[339] was a centre of pilgrimage by sick people.

Some Arabic authors from the 9th century mention traces of a temple at Memphis where miraculous cures were made and at its front a statue of a seated 'wise' man was to be seen and his wisdom was inscribed in the stela between his knees.[340]

The School of Alexandria

Titus Flavius Clemens (known as Clement of Alexandria, 150-215) describes the procession of the priests who carried 42 sacred books thought to have been written originally by Thoth/Hermes and containing hymns to the gods and the king which were kept in the temples. Four of them were about astronomy, ten about ceremonies and ten others about the gods and the education of priests; but six of them were dedicated to medicine covering: anatomy, surgery, ophthalmology, gynaecology and therapeutics. The fact that these books were known at Alexandria in the third century reflects the knowledge of ancient Egyptians in the scientific tradition of Alexandria during the Ptolemaic period. It was said that they were written by Horus Djer, king of the Ist Dynasty, but they were never found.

Hippocrates of Cos, (c. 460 a. C-c. 370 a. C), author of the *Corpus Hippocratum* containing medical texts from this school, compiled at Alexandria in the Second century BC, could have been the author of all the texts but there is no evidence for it, as some of the texts could have been written by his disciples. Soranus of Ephesus, a Greek gynaecologist from the Second century, was his first biographer and the source for much of the knowledge we have about him. Also Aristotelis wrote about him, in the 4th century BC

Soranus says that the father of Hippocrates was Heraclides, doctor; and that his sons, Tessalo and Draco, and his step son, Polybius, were his disciples. Galen says that Polybius was the successor of Hippocrates. His therapeutic theory was based in the curative power of nature (*vis medicatrix naturae*) and the body was the balance of the four humours, each person must heal his own self (*physis*).[341]

The existence of Egyptian doctors teaching at Alexandria and also embalmers with the knowledge of anatomy, has contributed to the development of medicine, revealing that Greek influence found support in the existing Egyptian tradition. Rufus de Ephesus, another doctor, was an important anatomist, as he described the tendons' glands, he studied cardiology and ophthalmology and he was known for his treatment by compression (Second century); and when he visited Egypt, he wrote that Egyptian doctors already gave names to cranial sutures although they barely understood Greek.

Asclepius of Bitinia implanted Greek medicine in the Roman kingdom in the first century BC. He opposed the humours' theory, defended by Egyptian medicine, as he thought that the body was composed of disconnected particles, or atoms, and separated by pores. Disease was caused by restriction of the movement needed by atoms or by blocked pores. Besides those doctors, there was also Galen from Pergamo, a Greek, and Paul of Egina, a Greek also, (625-690 BC) working at Alexandria; who wrote *Epítome of Medicine*, in seven books based on Hippocratic texts. These two had the method of drugs by grades, based on humours. Also Aulus Cornelius Celsus, a Roman, wrote an encyclopaedia of medicine; the Greek Pedanius Dioscorides (fl. 50-70), o first scientific botanic, that, in his *Materia Medica* classifies the prescriptions according to its effects on the patients.

In Greco-Roman Egypt doctors offered their services to everyone who asked for them; they were even exempted from participation in religious ceremonies. But this exemption was given by special privilege; some did not get it and they complained about it when they were called. They would have to make evidence of their profession to the *strategos* – the administrative officer – that they were established as doctors. As there was no system to licence the medical practice in Antiquity, Flavius Claudius Julianus, known also as Julian the Apostate (331 or 332 – 363), the Roman Emperor, commands the end of teaching by non-authorized people in 362 and, in the legislation of the IVth and 5th century more prerogative and immunities are extended to doctors.[342]

When the Arabs arrived in Egypt in 642, there was still a school of medicine that was active in Alexandria, where Syriac was spoken, and where many students, from the Middle East, were learning. Following the invasion of Byzantine Alexandria by the Arabs, many books were translated to Arabic. They were the ones allowing large advancements in medicine, judged and prohibited by the Catholic Church in their transposition to the West. Only after the Renaissance and still censured by the Inquisition, these books became known by all doctors in the West, with their innovative approaches and concepts, so well known today, such as the ones dealing with sexuality, one example of this is by the Portuguese Amato Lusitano.[343] The Egyptian pharmacopoeia from the pharaonic era which continued to be used in the Greco-Roman period was known by all populations in Antiquity and was used throughout the middle Ages with minor adaptations, until the XVIII century, and it is being rediscovered today.

---

[339] The Museum of Imhotep at Saqqara was opened in April, 2006.
[340] Nagy, 1999: 81.
[341] E. Littré, *Oeuvres complètes d'Hippocrate*, 10 volumes, Paris, Baillière, em http://www.bium.univ-paris5.fr

[342] Lewis, 1965: 91.
[343] Firmino Crespo: Lusitano, Amato, *Centúrias de Curas Medicinais,* Universidade New de Lisboa, 1980 and some recent articles upon his *Centúrias* at: Cadernos de Cultura da Universidade da Beira Interior da Covilhã: http://historiadamedicina.ubi.pt/cadernos.html

Anatomy

" (...) *in treatment, the anatomical knowledge applied was taken from earlier medical observations and theories, not from the science of mummification. (...).*"[344]
There are about 250 anatomical words in ancient Egyptian; either from the butcher shop or the embalmer's, using in the majority of cases characters representing animal physiology (mammals). They also used non-human names to describe body parts or actions performed by the human body in ancient Egypt. Anatomical words in hieroglyphic writing state that form precedes function; meaning, that words describing form are more important in the illustration of the organ, part of the body or its consistency than its function as a human organism. The body was seen as an ensemble of distinctive parts and its division was made more for the region of the body itself than by its function as we do today. Each region assembled the organs, muscles, tendons, substances flowing in that region, its *liaisons* (channels and articulations). An articulation was seen by ancient Egyptians as a separating line more than a connection between two parts. In hieroglyphic writing signs were used to show back and front also.

Some words regarding medical aspects and body parts in ancient Egyptian:

Doctor – *sunu*

swnw

Pill[345] – *suit*

swit

Prescription or medicine[346] – *pekheret*

pḫrt

Skull[347] – *djennet*

ḏnnt

Brain[348] - *amem*

ꜥmm

Nose[349] – *fenedj*

fnḏ

Mouth[350] – *er*

er

Ear[351] – *medjer*

mḏr

Eye[352] – *iret*

irt

Tooth – *ibeh*

ibḥ

Stomach[353] (mouth of the heart) – *ra-ib*

r- ib

Heart[354] – *ib ou haty*

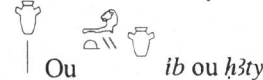

Ou   *ib ou ḥꜣty*

Lungs[355] – *sema*

smꜣ

Back bone (vertebral column) – *iat*

iꜣt

Womb/abdomen/belly[356] – *het*

ḥt

Stomach[357] – *mendjer*

mnḏr

Liver[358] –*miset*

mist

Mist[359]

mist

Spleen[360] - *nenechem*

nnšm

Gall bladder[361] – *weded*

[344] Győry, 2006: 2.
[345] Walker, 1996: 231.
[346] Nunn, 1996: 223.
[347] Nunn, 1996: 219; Ebeid, 1999: 96.
[348] Ebeid, 1999: 96.
[349] Ebeid, 1999: 96; Lisboa, 1978: 281.
[350] Lisboa, 1978: 282.

[351] Ebeid, 1999: 96.
[352] Ebeid, 1999: 96; Lisboa, 1978: 281.
[353] Ebeid, 1999: 97; Nunn, 1996: 46.
[354] Ebeid, 1999: 97.
[355] Ebeid, 1999: 97.
[356] Walker, 1996: 290; Nunn, 1996: 222; Gardiner F32, ideogram of animal womb, Gardiner, 2005: 464.
[357] Walker, 1996: 213.
[358] Walker, 1996: 302; Ebeid, 1999: 97; Nunn, 1996: 46.
[359] Walker, 1996: 297.
[360] Walker, 1996: 338,339; Ebeid, 1999: 97
[361] Ebeid, 1999: 97; Nunn, 1996: 46.

wdd

Bile[362] – *benef*

bnf

Intestines[363] – *mehetu*

mḫt

qab[364]

k3b

Bladder[365] – *cheptit*

šptyt

Uterus – *idet*[366]

hemet[367]

ḥmt

Pelvis[368] – *peheui*

pḥwi

Anus[369] – *aret*

'rt

Kidneys[370] – *geget*

ggt

Skin[371] – *inem*

inm

Channels/vessels[372] – *metu*

mt

Pus[373] – *rit*

ryt

Sweat[374] – *fedet*

fdt

Menstruation[375] – *hesmen*

ḥsmn

The Per-Ankh, a Hospital-School?

The medical teaching was done in the "Houses of Life"; Gardiner says that these were the locations where scribes copied ancient texts. A doctor from Ramesses II reign says: "I was formed in the school of medicine of Heliopolis where (...) I was taught (...) medicines. I was formed in the gynaecological school of Sais, where divine hands gave me their recipes. I have all the spells personally prepared by Osiris. MY guide was always the god Thoth, inwindr of speech and author of infallible recipes, the only one who knows how to give magicians a reputation[376] and to doctors that follow his perceptions. The spells are excellent medicines and the medicines are good spells".[377]

"(...) The magician performing the rite and the individual who believes in it".[378]

The Per-Ankh or House of Life was the Library where scientific records were kept and where priests learned their duties, future scribes learned written hieroglyphic, religious concepts, scientific and cultural thoughts of ancient Egypt.[379]

Large collections of books were kept in these Houses as is attested by Galen in his *De composit medicament*, V, 2.[380] It was also here that dreams were interpreted, a divination procedure practised in ancient Egypt.[381]

The teaching of medicine was done by the Papyri and animal dissection. Only in the Ptolemaic period human cadavers are examined, not before. The medical school at the temple of Zau, Sais in Greek, and Sa el-Hagar in Arabic is well recorded.[382] Besides centres of teaching, This 'Houses' were the place where medical Papyri were written (copied) and kept.

---

[362] Nunn, 1996: 218. Bile as ingredient in medical prescriptions.
[363] Walker, 1996: 313.
[364] Ebeid, 1999: 97.
[365] Ebeid, 1999: 98.
[366] Nunn, 1996: 47
[367] Ebeid, 1999: 97;
[368] Walker, 1996: 334.
[369] Walker, 1996: 247.
[370] Walker, 1996: 278
[371] Ebeid, 1999: 97; Lisboa, 1978: 281. In this word the last hieroglyph can be hair , Gardiner D3, or the leather from the cow' skin , Gardiner F27, as shown here.
[372] Faulkner, 2006: 120.

[373] Nunn, 1996: 224.
[374] Nunn, 1996: 219; Lisboa, 1978: 281.
[375] Nunn, 1996: 221.
[376] A magician invokes and uses the power: Meyer, Smith, 1994: 5.
[377] Lisboa, 1978: 283.
[378] Claude Lévi-Strauss quoted in Meyer, Smith, 1994: 6.
[379] Nunn, 1996: 131; Ghalioungui, 1963: 42.
[380] Ghalioungui, 1963: 42.
[381] Ghalioungui, 1963: 43.
[382] Cuenca-Estrella, 2004: 60.

In an Egyptian ritual described in *Papyrus Salt* 825, BM 10051, for the protection of the Per-Ankh, the sacred precinct of Osiris' temple at Abydos, the conservation of a mummy must be assured, representing Osiris and Ra together, in the interior of the House of Life; describing endless enemies and stating that the mummy represents Life, therefore ensuring that the Sun continues its course.[383] The text in this papyrus prescribes instructions for the ceremony of protection, forbidding the entry of enemies by manufacturing wax figures.[384]

An inscription on a statue from a doctor, of the 6th century BC, from Sais, tells of the Persian king Dario who ordered this doctor to refurbish the Houses of Life at Sais and other locations. In the first millennium BC, at Sais as in Bubastis these Houses were well known to Egyptians.[385]

Since the Ist Dynasty, (c. 3150-2925 BC), Per-Ankh are recorded to have existed. Of all, the one with the better reputation was the one from Imhotep at Memphis which had an international reputation, especially because of its' Library which existed until the first years of the Christian era. Also, the one at Sais which trained midwives who taught themselves their art of doctors (obstetrics) and also the Per-Ankh of Abydos where Ramesses IV frequently visited its' Library.[386]

At least four Houses of Life were connected to temples at Bubastis, Edfu, Amarna and Kom Ombo. Medicine would have been more secular in the Old Kingdom and during large part of Middle Kingdom, but gradually became more mystical at the hands of priests and exorcists, maybe because of the ascending political power of these priests in the New Kingdom, who tried to monopolize all branches of knowledge.

Also, it is a fact that more recent medical Papyri are basically magical while ancient papyri have less spells.

Instruments

Ancient Egyptian texts do not mention descriptions of instruments.[387] There are some items that have survived art depictions and some medical papyri that refer to which type of 'knife' was used for a specific prescription.

Knives used in medical acts had stone blades and sharpened edges that were sharper than surgical steel today, later on doctors used bronze blades and then iron blades as well. The cauterizing act accompanied the procedure, the blade was heated until it became incandescent and then it was used to make incisions, cutting and sealing the blood channels limiting the bleeding.

To cut the flesh they used the *ds* (Ebers 875), *ḥpt* (Ebers 767), *š3s* (Ebers 875), *psškf* or *swt* that had their characteristic shapes and sizes.[388]

At the Museum of History of Medicine in Paris there are some medical instruments from ancient Egypt brought by Clot Bei.[389]

In the temple dedicated to Haroeris at Kom Ombo, there is a relief of what seems to be a collection of 37 medical instruments: bone saws, suction glasses, knives, scalpels, retractors, scales, lancets and dental tools. Some of the instruments are difficult to identify as to what function they were designed for. Some of those can be ritual instruments.

The point is, what type of instruments would originally be Egyptian and what would be an 'import' from the Greeks or the Romans. We have to be cautious (in the attempt to identify and categorize) as cosmetic instruments, mummification, medical and even domestic instruments, could have been the same.[390]

The first specimen of scissors,[391] as we may call it, was invented c. 1500 BC and found in some ruins from ancient Egypt. This was a simple piece of metal, completely different from the ones we use today. Trepanation, practised in many cultures, is not mentioned in the medical Papyri but it seems to have been practised occasionally. Only fourteen skulls, with total or partial cures of the trepanning wound were found, and it is thought that amputations from limbs were also undertaken. "Sir Flinders Petrie describes the development of crossed blades from the first century. In the same century, the chronicler Isidore of Seville describes crossed blades or scissors as tools from the barber and the tailor. "[392]

O *pesechkef*, a prehistoric silex knife with a shape of a fish tail[393] is similar to the hairdressing knife of the goddess Meskhenet,[394] this knife was used as an essential instrument at the funerary ceremony of the Opening of the Mouth. In this ritual the mummy is reborn and recovers all the faculties and body functions that she/he would have had in life. There was a set of objects associated to this ritual as well as knives, small fluid containers that helped restore life, with milk (the first

---

[383] Derchain, 1959: 76-77.

[384] Ritner, 1993: 185; Kakosy, Roccati, 1999: 127.

[385] Pinch,1994: 63.

[386]Australian Academy of Medicine and Surgery: http://www.aams.org.au/contents.php?subdir=library/history/&filename =pharonic_egypt

[387] Györy, 2006: 1.

[388] Györy, 2006: 1.

[389] Musée de l'Histoire de la Médicine de Paris: http://www.bium.univ-paris5.fr/musee/

[390] Györy, 2006: 2.

[391] Ebeid, 1999: 130.

[392] Wiss, 1948.

[393] Nunn, 1996: 165.

[394] Birth goddess present at the Judgement so that the deceased can be 'reborn'.

nutrition received in life), salt water for cleansing and purification and sweet water.[395]

It was initially designed to cut the umbilical cord at birth,[396] approximately since c. 5000 BC[397] the *pesechkef*, performed for the deceased the magical moment of returning to life. According to E.O. Faulkner [398] *pesechkef* comes from the gathering of two words: *pesesh* — × meaning separation technique and *kef* , to discover, to denude and to undress. Therefore, its meaning is: the instrument to separate the flesh. In the rebirth scene from the *Papyrus of Ani* (British Museum 10470) there is a complete manual of survival for the afterlife.

Present at the Final Judgement to observe and secure the success of this task are the important gods associated with birth and destiny: Meskhenet[399] and Renenutet, goddess of breastfeeding. The *pesechkef* possibly represented the imaginary umbilical cord[400] and at some stage of the ritual, the funerary *sem* priest touched the mummy with this instrument, symbolizing the scene of his/her birth. Regarding Meskhenet, the knife that cuts the umbilical cord symbolizes the goddess of birth. But the hairdressing of Meskhenet can also be identified with a cow's uterus, in an allusion to Hathor, protector of maternity. An author has a different identification of *pesechkef* regarding the hairdressing of Meskhenet;[401] stating that this could have represented two stems of a plant.

2.2. Written magic

Written magic had a secret sense and code; it was a well kept secret by those practising it.

Many spells were written in the verso of Papyri showing letters and texts of myths and legends that were kept in the tomb with the deceased.[402] Some mix medical texts and magical ones. Between c. 2000 and 1150 BC the majority of texts found next to Egyptian mummified bodies were about pregnancy problems. And, to recite a spell out loud or to write it down was considered a magical act. As words were taken as divine, whether written or recited out loud, these should be treated with much respect. To know the name of something or someone meant to have power over it/the person.
Also the power of the word could be used with bad intentions, the imitation of names or the use of metaphors was a dangerous action.

All the ingredients used had usually strange names so that the common 'mortal' could not understand them nor copy them (punts).[403]

Gardiner suggests several of these 'semantic punts' *a propos* of several diseases.[404] Borghouts refers to some in magical texts (spell for the head).[405] There were words, 'punts' (sounding alike but having diverse meanings), that could mean different or opposite things and these were used as code in magic by who was able to decipher them and understand the subliminal message.

Examples: *remedj* – men, *remit* – tears from the Sun god; *benet* – harp, evil that is going to happen. An example pointed by Gardiner is the punt used in the interpretation of dreams as divination of the future that plays with words such as crocodile and officer comparing their greediness.[406] Another suggests that the association of, being on top of a sycamore tree, *nehat*, is a synonym of being well in life, *nehi*.[407] Sculptures, reliefs and images represented the essence of magic as shown in the sandals' drawing of king Tutankhamun stepping on the enemies, meaning that he had power over them.

The scenes of judgement of the deceased in funerary papyri had the future in them; names were the essence of the person; to erase the name of someone meant to erase his/her existence forever…The cartouche with the king's name was his essence having his magician knot.

Spells could be deposited in a basin and rinsed with water; the patient drank the water or threw it over the wound (ex.: the use of Horus' *cippus* to heal of snake or scorpion bite).[408] The power of healing the venom of a snake or scorpion consisted in washing the letters of the text written in the stela (*cippus*).[409]

Spells were also were written in myrrh ink, rinsed with spring water and then drank. Or they were written in the hand of the patient and licked by him/her. Spells started many times with the invocation of myths of divinities related to the specific cure. They were repeated several times. The magician tried to negotiate with the divinity or to trick it so it would leave the person. Dreams were much used as a vehicle for a spell.[410] In the New Kingdom Papyri compiled by Christian Leitzs' edition,[411] numerous magic spells and prayers against snake bites

---

[395] Allen, 2005: 28.
[396] Pinch, 1994: 130; Győry, 2006: 1.
[397] Harer, 1994: 1053; Nunn, 1996: 165.
[398] *The Ancient Egyptian Coffin Texts*, 1994.
[399] Protective goddess of newborns, represented with two bricks identifying the support where women gave birth; also connected to the deceased 'rebirth', helping Isis and Nephtys.
[400] Szpakowska, 2006: 57.
[401] Castel, 2004, http://www.Egyptlogia.com/content/view/462/73/
[402] Ritner, 1993: 180-183.
[403] Scott Noegel, assistant professor of Languages and Civilizations of Near East at the University of Washington, Seattle, USA studies punts in ancient Egyptian literature, regarding dream interpretation: *Nocturnal Ciphers: The Punning Language of Dreams in the Ancient Near East*, American Oriental Series 89, New Haven, Connecticut, American Oriental Society, 2007; Meyer e Smith, 1994: 14.
[404] Szpakowska, 2003: 81-85; 89, 95, 102, 104, 107-108, 111, 129, 132, 149.
[405] Borghouts, 1978: 32.
[406] Szpakowska, 2003: 82.
[407] Szpakowska, 2003: 82, 84.
[408] Borghouts, 1978: 59, 62, 69, 83; Pinch, 1994: 134.
[409] Meyer, Smith, 1994: 80.
[410] Pinch, 1994: 160.
[411] Leitz, 1999.

can be read. In the *Harris Papyrus* it is said that perfect spells should be sung, with a refrain and everything. The majority of those spells were intended to cast away crocodiles.[412]

Sekhmet e Mut

Sekhmet is usually portrayed with a human female body and the head of a lioness and as the daughter of the sun god, Ra with a solar disc and the *uraeus* in her head.[413] This represented her intimate relationship with Uraeus or Uadjit, in her role of fire spitter, impersonating the eye of Ra[414] (as Sekhmet, Tefnut or Mehit)[415] holding the *ankh* of life in her left hand.[416]

The name of Sekhmet means literally "The Powerful".[417] Sekhmet embodies the female aggressive side and acts as consort of Ptah.[418] Some statues were placed in several Museums such as the Metropolitan Museum of Art of New York and Turin Egyptian Museum; all are part of a bigger group of seven hundred statues ordered by Amenhotep III.[419]

She is the patron of medicine by excellence in ancient Egypt. The Pyramid Texts mention that the king would have been conceived by her, Sekhmet; therefore she is seen as the divine mother of kings and the god Khonsu.
Her name and power derive from the word, in ancient Egyptian, *sekhem*, which means power or powerful. Sekhmet was worshipped over all Upper Egypt, especially where an oasis was growing in the desert.[420]

This is the type of ground where lionesses are found abundantly[421] as they come from the interior of the desert to drink and then stay and hang around the location, waiting for prey. Both the *Ebers Papyrus* and the *Edwin Smith Papyrus* do not seem to make any large distinction between the work of the *sunu* and the work of the *uab* priest of Sekhmet in diagnosing diseases.[422]

Her cult was based in Memphis and was part of the divine triad: Ptah, Sekhmet and Nefertum. Due to the change of power from Memphis to Thebes in the New Kingdom (1550- 1069 BC) and the existence of a new triad to be worshipped, Amun, Mut and Khonsu, Sekhmet syncretised with Mut[423] representing jointly the aggressive manifestation of Mut[424] and the soft form of Bastet.[425] Mut-Sekhmet was the "royal protector, Wife of the King of Gods, The One Who Incarnated in the Person of the Pharaoh". When she destroys it is always fitting; it had to happen or a vengeance was necessary. Never by chance as she punishes whoever disregards the rules of Maat.

Isis cures his son, Horus, with an amulet of Sekhmet.[426]

At the precinct of Mut at Karnak numerous statues of Sekhmet are being dug out of the ground;[427] at the location where a temple was ordered to be built by Amenhotep III (1390 - 1352 BC),[428] maybe many of those were brought from another previous building located near the Colossi of Memnon. It is thought today that the Sekhmet statues carrying the name of Amenhotep III would have been originally created for his funerary temple in the western bank of the Nile. Some might have been transported to Mut's precinct during the XIXth Dynasty when Mut and Sekhmet were associated and rituals were common in the sacred lake, *isheru*.[429]

There were priests and shrines dedicated to her in Lower Egypt, at Memphis, as she was the patron of disease and cure; she was also able to inflict death and disease. There is a text that describes the fear of Sekhmet which spread between the people in times of plague which states when priests should intervene in favour of whom she punished.[430]

The Lady of Life, the Powerful, the force that fought the diseases! As god-that-heals, Sekhmet had the power to destroy and she was invoked against invisible demons of plagues and diseases; the priests of Sekhmet were trained surgeons, of excellent reputation, according to the scientific patterns of antiquity, fighting priests, scorpion charmers, and scribes at the House of Life. These priests of Sekhmet were able to make diseases go back to their origin, so believed the ancient Egyptians and therefore deposit all hope in these priests when nothing else prevailed. Priests of Sekhmet, *uab sekhmet*, knew how to calm her wrath and how to transform her into a benevolent goddess. They formed a society of healers using magical procedures to fight against plagues in Egypt.[431]

---

[412] Chabas, X: 139.
[413] Ebeid, 1999: 375.
[414] Lichtheim, 1997: 36.
[415] Nagy, 1999: 74.
[416] Allen, 2005: 47.
[417] McClung Museum, The University of Tennessee, Knoxville, Tennessee, USA, http://mcclungMuseumm.utk.edu/specex/scholars/scholars.htm
[418] Sales, 1999: 283; Dicionário do Ancient Egypt, 2001: 772.
[419] Allen, 2005: 47.
[420] A variation of Sekhmet, Mehit, and a lioness goddess identified with Tefnut, wife of Shu and also ichnographically represented as a woman with a lioness head.
[421] Sales, 1999: 287.
[422] Nunn, 1996: 134-135.
[423] Germond, 2005: 36.

[424] Pinkowski, Jennifer, *Egypt's Ageless Goddess*, Archaeology, Volume 59 Number 5, September/October 2006, http://www.archaeology.org/0609/abstracts/mut.html
[425] "In the temple of Koptos, the goddess Mut of Thebes was called sometimes Bast and other times Sekhmet of Memphis", Erman, Adolf, *A Handbook of Egyptian Religion*, 1907: 56 quoting Petrie, W.M. Flinders, *Koptos*, D.G. Hogarth, London, 1896.
[426] Borghouts, 1978: 85-86.
[427] JHU Expedition, Mut Temple Precinct, http://www.jhu.edu/~neareast/egypttoday.html; Brooklyn Museum: Dig Diary, http://digdiary.blogspot.com/
[428] Pinch, 1994: 143.
[429] The sacred lake from the temple of Mut at Karnak, a John Hopkins University's excavation project.
[430] Ebeid, 1999: 72.
[431] Sales, 1999: 284.

A code of ethics was followed and an oath was probably given by doctors.

Beer is connected to the myth of Sekhmet, maybe originating at festivals performed after the battles. The myth tells of how she was created from the eye of Ra to destroy humankind, she gets drunk, but Ra gives her beer with red ochre to look like blood to make her cease the bloody killing, and so she gives it up. At the tomb of Niankhsekhmet, from the Vth Dynasty, was written: "Never did anything evil to any person", a type of Hippocratic Oath.[432]

Personal practices

There were several ways of administering medical remedies; oral, rectal, vaginal and topical, by fumigation and in methods of administration: pills, cakes, suppositories, unguents, drops, mouth washes and baths. The fluids in which the medicine was contained were also varied: water, milk, mucus, beer and wine, always sweetened with honey or dates.[433]
The king was also considered divine, therefore all his body parts and fluids were believed to have magical powers. Manicurists and hairdressers from the king had a special high social status as it was their responsibility to ensure the safety of the physical remains (hair and nails) from the king so that it would not be used against him.

Another example of magical reinforcement was the painting of the eye udjat, wḏȝt, in the hand with ochre for protection with the name of the person before reciting the magical formula. This was the procedure for the treatment of a patient: the magician comes to the person or the patient was brought to the presence of the magician executing the spell/medicine. After some preparation and purification of the location, the magical words were spoken and the rituals[434] executed. The majority of patients would not feel an immediate recovery and therefore they wanted to retain the magical force with them so that it would act on them for much longer.

Ritual texts were not abstract or limited to a mere recitation, but they involved a broader choice of practices frequently described within them. These texts were answers to the requirements of each person in times of crisis, pain, travel and specific problems of daily life.[435] Many texts were spells to cure or protect from disease.[436]

So everyone carried an object of a protective nature, an amulet. An afflicted person could ask an oracle which divinity he/she had offended so that the prayer would be more effective or the spell best designed for the cure.

The headrests, of which we have many specimens in museums today, usually had some inscriptions of gods in its' base and also in the headrest itself (the part where the head is supported) to cast away evils spirits.

People were often buried with amulet-papyri[437] which they used in life as amulets. Their texts were written in such a way that they seemed like divine. They listed the body parts of the patient and they secured immunity to the querent.[438] The person was identified in it as being the main character in the myth and transferred his/her problem from human to the gods' sphere so that cosmic forces such as heka could be used to solve the matter.

Ancient Egyptians thought that to bury magical objects[439] and ingredients used in spells, even the remains and waste, perpetuated the power of the spell.

2.3. Amulets

Could be made by man or nature; stones, sea shells, nature oddities and especially those presenting odd shapes were considered special, in particular if those shapes were reminders of human genitals. Amulets in ancient Egypt date from c. 4000 BC, and magical texts date from approx. 3000 BC until 500 AD. The number of amulets is put at 275, but this is probably underestimated; there would have been many more.[440] The ones found in tombs were maybe those which the deceased had used in life to ensure his/her protection. They were too personal to be left for anyone else.[441]

Amulets that were integrated in spells were similar to the forces of nature; the waters of the Nile that could not flood the land; the Sun cycle that may not be completed; therefore the magician speaks as if he was god. But not all amulets were buried with the deceased to protect him/her in the afterlife or to protect a person whilst alive; there were also temporary amulets for childbirth, disease or travel purposes.[442]

Children were highly protected beings as they were more vulnerable to diseases and danger. Also it was thought that spirits from deceased women (women that would have died from childbirth), or women without children were envious of new lives, therefore much feared by children and their mothers.[443] In many tombs containing infant bodies amulets were found: necklaces of pearls, corals or sea shells, the majority of objects being toys. These were manufactured by the father, or bought. The female figurines found reveal that they are not always of erotic intent as in the context of child death there is a doll or a figurine showing the sexual organs naked as a

---

[432] Sameh, 2006.
[433] Sipos, Gyory, Hagymási, Onderjka, Blázovics, 2004: 212.
[434] Rituals have a social function but some seem to be, private activities that were performed in secret: Meyer, Smith, 1994: 5.
[435] Meyer, Smith, 1994: 14.
[436] Meyer, Smith, 1994: 29.

[437] Examples at the Turin, London, Paris, Berlin, Cairo, New York, Philadelphia and Chicago Museum.
[438] Kakosy, Roccati, 1991: 118.
[439] Ritner, 1993: 172-179.
[440] Pinch, 1994: 105.
[441] Pinch, 1994: 104.
[442] Pinch, 1994: 105.
[443] Pinch, 1994: 123, 149.

promise of fertility and prosperity associated with the afterlife.

Since c. 1000 BC the Moon becomes more important in ancient Egyptian beliefs; the civil calendar is based on Moon phases[444] restricted to the religious functions in the temple;[445] the dawn was the better hour to perform spells and prayers as it is the time of cosmic renewal. The inscriptions from Edfu show both the civil calendar and the calendar based on Moon phases.[446]

One curiosity is the use of human ears as amulets on prayers made to divinities. This is aimed at turning divinities into 'large' listeners of human prayers. The crucial importance of the ear was because it was through the right ear that gods conceded life and though the left ear that they took life. The amputation was a serious punishment bearing this belief in mind.[447] Although the bovine ear was used as an ideogram in written hieroglyphics, the human ear was used in prayers. Some divinities are called listeners or large listeners.[448] During the New Kingdom votive stelae bearing large ears were used by those who decided to discard a priest for the prayer using human ears attributed to some divinities being asked for blessings and that were considered magic.

Some words used for personal protection:[449]

Amulets or spells to protect: *udjau,* *wḏȝw,* from *udjat,* *wḏȝt,* the eye of Horus, a protector.

sa, , meant amulet *sȝ* and protection *sȝw,* the word *sa* may mean a group of objects that are 'tied'; a rope that ties them down; the bag (tied) with the contents of an amulet and the words and gestures necessary to activate the spell.[450]

sau, magician *sȝw*

nehet, prayer *nḥt,* the hieroglyph used here is the binding element; knots had a special importance in tying the prayer, and they are still used today in magic of African influence; afro-American (south USA and Caribbean) and Arabic (North Africa).[451]

nedj, ask for advice , *nḏ*

meket, support/protection , *mkt*

mki, to protect, guard , *mki*

mek, protector , *mk*

Some doctors had this title, *sau* (from *sa,* protection), they practiced medicine and they were sometimes the "man-amulet". In this designation were included those that manufactured the amulets and those that read spells. There was also the denomination for women *sau*; a wooden figurine found in the X7th century BC is one of these fighters against demons, Beset. She uses a mask of a leonine demon and two wands in her hands in the shape of snakes. It was found in a tomb under the Ramesseum at Thebes[452]

The *sa* was a visual representation of a protection concept, much used in amulets[453] as magical wands [454] and jewellery, in the hope of giving protection to the wearer and it was also a component of other amulets such as the *ankh, djed* and *uas.*

The *udjat* eye, *wḏȝt* of Horus was a strong amulet, of an essentially protective charge. It can be represented by a shepherd's rope or the papyrus rolled by barge men in the Nile. This hieroglyph is shown in two ways; in the Old Kingdom, the lower part of the rope was not divided, in Middle Kingdom the end of the rope is shown usually separated. As the eye of Horus was torn out by Seth when fighting and then restored by Thoth (he was integrated again, *udjat,* united)[455] it is used as protection in doors, tombs and over the incision made in the human body to remove the organs before embalming the body ensuring its' protection.

This myth of the *udjat* eye was probably used as an attempt to recreate the myth of the Contendings between Horus e Seth, found in a group of manuscripts from Deir el-Medina; in the *Papyrus Chester Beatty* I, the sole copy of this myth, preserved in Dublin.[456] The Contendings between Horus and Seth represents the classic of the war between Good and Evil. The *udjat* eye, the right eye of Horus, represents the Sun, the god Ra, and the male side. The left eye represents the Moon,[457] and the god Thoth, god of magic, the female side, and can explain the connection with the phases of the moon during the month (lunar month, 28 days).

Since the end of Old Kingdom, *udjat* eyes were sometimes painted in sarcophagi so that the deceased could see through them.[458] The apotropaic function of the eye was described in the Egyptian texts as a protection against the evil-eye, so well known today.[459] The eye of

---

[444] Twelve months of thirty days and five epagomenal days, receding in time in comparison with the solar calendar to the reason of one day in each four years, as it is a quarter of day shorter than the solar year, Depuydt, 1997:270
[445] Depuydt, 1997: 138-140.
[446] Depuydt, 1997: 220.
[447] *En Egypte antique,* 2005.
[448] Ebeid, 1999: 86.
[449] Words in ancient Egyptian, Faulkner, 2006.
[450] Pinch, 1994: 108.
[451] Presentation shown by Remke Kruk at a lecture in *Ritual Healing,* Warburg Institute, London, February 2006. Remke Kruk is a lecturer at the Leiden University in literature, philosophy, and Arabic science and religion: http://www.cnws.leidenuniv.nl/index.php3-c=430.htm

[452] Pinch, 1994: 56-57.
[453] Russmann, 2001: 110.
[454] Pinch, 1994: 79.
[455] Kakosy, Roccati, 1999:82
[456] Chester Beatty Library, Dublin: http://www.cbl.ie/Collections/The-Western-Collection/Papyri/Egyptian.aspx
[457] Explained by the ancient Egyptians, unique events such as solar and lunar eclipses as being the two eyes of the divinity, Kakosy, Roccati, 1999: 82; Pinch, 1994: 27.
[458] Kakosy, Roccati, 1999: 84.
[459] Kakosy, Roccati, 1999: 84.

Horus, besides its' protective and healing powers as an amulet was also used as a unit for measurement in medicine, general accounting and measuring cereals where it determined the ingredients' proportions to use.

The magical wands were inspired by the wooden sticks thrown to birds as having a type of sign of control from the magician over all demons;[460] also called apotropaic, meaning 'something that casts away evil'. They were made of hippopotamus' ivory and the oldest ones date from c. 2800 BC,[461] examples previous to the XIIth Dynasty are not known, according to Éva Liptay from the Museum of Fine Arts in Budapest.[462]

They would be used to draw a protective circle in the ground around the person asking for protection. Therefore, some show the tips worn and also fissures from accidental breakings. These wands were inscribed with evil beings invoked by magicians to fight in defence of the afflicted person. Many present the magicians fighting creatures or demons as *sau*, the protectors, *aha*, and *netjeru*, gods.[463] These magicians are shown stabbing, squeezing or biting evil forces; which are represented by snakes and foreigners. Some wands had hands carved in their tips as representations of the act of sealing the spell and some are made in the shape of hands.

The *aha* were fighting demons carved in wands used mainly by ordinary people, with no access to temples, limited spaces to priests, but these limitations tend to disappear with time, and therefore temples become more accessible to the general population c.1600 BC.

From the first millennium BC and during the Roman period a type of disc was placed under the head of the deceased and these discs were called hypocephali (from the Greek *hypokephalos*, under the head, a translation of the Egyptian *hr tp* with the same meaning). These objects were made in the shape of a small disc and the materials used for its' manufacture range from papyrus, stuccoed linen, bronze, gold, wood, or clay. The hypocephalus represented all that the sun encircles, its upper portion represented the world of men and the day sky, and the lower portion (the part with the cow) the nether world and the night sky.[464] Its' function was, according to chapter 162 from The Book of The Dead, to allow the deceased to feel the heat of the Sun god Amun-Ra.[465]

The spell around the outside of the disc is an abbreviated form of Chapter 162: *'Cause to come into being a flame*

beneath his head for he is the soul of that corpse which rests in Heliopolis, Atum is his name'.[466] The headrests were also powerful amulets, protecting the thoughts and dreams of its owner while he/she rested in life or death. They were used until the Ptolemaic period.[467]

In the Book of The Dead there is a chapter dedicated to the headrest, chapter 166, where the deceased is considered a sleeping patient whose head needs to be elevated to the horizon of Amun.[468]

So, as the Sun was reborn everyday so the deceased could also be reborn. The god Bes, protector of children, is very frequently represented in these headrests,[469] with his menacing features to cast away evil spirits.

The number seven was a magic number.[470] The 11th line in the protection against evil-eye had seven *udjat* eyes to be effective in the interruption of evil actions.[471]

An example of this is a wooden table from c. 400 BC, with an inscription for protection. On its right hand side it has seven *udjat* eyes and Ptah, Min, Thoth, Horus, Isis and Nephtys figures.

The amulets used in ancient Egypt were classified by Flinders Petrie as belonging to several categories, relevant for their connection to medicine; homeopathic, prophylactic and theomorphic.[472]

Homeopathic,[473] those where the animal physical characteristics were transferred to the human; prophylactic (protection: Bes, Taweret, Udjat or repellent: from crocodiles and scorpions) the ones that give protection for or against, to the person and theomorphic (amulets covering all gods with relevance for health according to the formulated wish).

The records of medical practices in Coptic Egypt show that lines between magic, medicine and religion that frequently are taken as present in our societies, did not exist for the people of those texts.[474]

Some Coptic amulets from the 4th century to the 8th century describe protections and treatments for personal health: *Berlin Papyrus* 21911 for eye treatments;[475] the ostracon of the Egger collection, in Paris, as an amulet to cure;[476] the *Parchment Oxyrhynchus* 1077 to cure (using a Christian text), Greek letters and a human figure in the

---

[460] Pinch, 1994: 40.
[461] Pinch, 1994: 40.
[462] *A propos* of the exhibition *Repelling Demon -Protecting Newborns* at the Museum of Fine Arts in Budapest, Oct, 21 to Nov, 20, 2005: http://ibisz.freeweb.hu/hun/hazai/kiallit/idoszak/kama2005a.html
[463] Pinch, 1994: 42.
[464] Rhodes, Michael D., *The Joseph Smith Hypocephalus Seventeen Years Later*, http://www.lightplanet.com/response/BofAbraham/jshypo.htm#fn5
[465] Kakosy, Roccati, 1999: 90.

[466] http://www.britishmuseum.org/explore/highlights/highlight_objects/aes/h/hypocephalus_of_the_temple_mus.aspx
[467] Russmann, 2001: 162.
[468] Faulkner, 1972 : 15 ; Trindade Lopes, 1991 : 247-48 ; *Toutankhamon et son temps*, 1967
[469] Russmann, 2001: 162.
[470] Pinch, 1994: 37.
[471] Kakosy, Roccati, 1999: 84.
[472] Nunn, 1996: 110.
[473] Nunn, 1996: 110.
[474] Meyer, Smith, 1994: 79.
[475] Meyer, Smith, 1994: 32.
[476] Meyer, Smith, 1994: 32.

centre;[477] the *Florence Papyrus* 365 at the Instituto de Papirologia G. Vitelli to cure a woman;[478] another for women's cures: the *Berlin Papyrus* 21230,[479] the *Oxyrhynchus Papyrus* 924,[480] the *Oxyrhynchus Papyrus* 1151,[481] the *Vienna Rainer Papyrus* 5 (13b)[482] and an amulet for a man, Silvanus, to grant him good health, folded and tied with a red string to be worn by him.[483]

In the *Vienna Papyrus* K8303, the text has 43 curative spells operating by two basic principles; the content of the spell brings power to its owner through contact with the letters and the inscribed spell represents its own perpetual recitation.[484]

The *Cairo Papyrus* 45060, found in a jar buried in a monastic cell, at Thebes, contains several prescriptions for the treatment of diverse diseases (ophthalmological, and gynaecological among others).

The *Michigan Papyrus* 593 has twenty pages, for physical and psychological ailments. Some of these prescriptions have references to the cooking of sympathetic elements that are ingested, taken in baths or applied as unguents. Some of these must have been placebos but others reveal a more scientific approach as curative balms and medicines.[485]

These prescriptions are organized like this: eighteen according to the affected body zone; abdominal problems (4-5), head (6-9), sleep (10-11), respiratory (14-15), central nervous system (17-18), breastfeeding (32), menstruation/bleedings (23).[486]

As actions to undertake were to wash, to drink, to annoint, to pour, to bind, to use or to eat and the organic means to use, water, olive oil, vinegar, peppermint, figs, wine, ibis' blood, marine salt and sweets in general.[487]

In a spell against a *samana* demon, describing the attacked body parts, there is a mention to the seven knots of the head[488] and the seven openings for the sensorial organs, according to Borghouts.[489]

Some examples of amulets:
Linen bandages with written magical words
A lock of hair with four knots tied to the throat
A fish spine in a string tied with a knot

Knots had special importance as it was believed that they could bind forces and thus be an obstacle to evil.[490]

Knots made of linen were temporary amulets and the ones made of jewellery were considered to grant eternal protection.[491]

There were inumerous amulets for different situations that will not be studied in detail for this work here, limiting the description to some of the more important found with several mummies and on excavation sites throughout the XIXth and XXth centuries.

As symbol of eternal prosperity ancient Egyptians used *djed pillar* symbolizing Osiris, of which both the hieroglyph and amulet refer to Osiris' vertebral column and to his resurrection; the knot of the Isis' *tyet* representing a buckle with knot, much used for conception, looking like an *ankh* with folded arms; the girdle or buckle of Isis, as it was also called. It may represent the menstrual blood flow from the womb of the god and its magical properties.[492]

The animal representing Seth was probably a desert animal that is now completely vanished from the Egyptian landscape, associated with all kinds of disturbances and as a determinative in hieroglyphic writing, it could be used to define climate change, aggression and any manifestation of power, noise and also details of medical prescriptions. If this animal did exist, it has been studied, but a question remains; the use of its ears and erect tail in texts or references reflect a predator, as god Seth. Words[493] that show this influence of the 'Sethian' determinative:

Disease, affliction/concern, *inedj* ind

To be ill, *mer* mr

To suffer, *nekem* nkm

In March 2006, the Egyptologist Salima Ikram, director of the project Animal Mummies at the Cairo Egyptian Museum, and also co-director of the North Kharga Oasis Survey,494 regarding some items found, said[495] "They're images of Seth and some mentions of Amun having to do with Seth as well. It also has a couple of other New Kingdom inscriptions relating to scribes that we haven't deciphered yet. Now, nobody knows what the Seth animal is. It's probably some kind of an amalgam of wild desert types. "

[477] Meyer, Smith, 1994: 33.
[478] Meyer, Smith, 1994: 38.
[479] Meyer, Smith, 1994: 38.
[480] Meyer, Smith, 1994: 39.
[481] Meyer, Smith, 1994: 40.
[482] Meyer, Smith, 1994: 41.
[483] Meyer, Smith, 1994: 42.
[484] Meyer, Smith, 1994: 81.
[485] Meyer, Smith, 1994: 298.
[486] Meyer, Smith, 1994: 299-300, 305-307.
[487] Meyer, Smith, 1994: 300.
[488] Borghouts, 1978: 81.
[489] Borghouts, 1978: 21.

[490] Pinch, 1994:108; Borghouts, 1978: 31.
[491] Pinch, 1994: 83, 108; Still today, in *Kabbalah*, Jewish belief of ancient times in the magic of words, a red string of virgin wool is used as protector from the evil eye, in the left wrist, the side where evil enters the body. Seven knots are given to the string reciting a prayer of seven lines (each line to a knot): http://www.kabbalah.com/13.php
[492] Pinch, 1994: 116.
[493] McDonald, 2000; 79; Faulkner, 2006: 24, 110.
[494] *North Kharga Oasis Survey*, American University of Cairo: http://www.aucegypt.edu/academic/northkhargaoasissurvey/home.html
[495] Ikram, 2006.

The scarab, *kheper*, was preferably made of stone and placed next to the heart of the deceased meaning to be reborn, to come back to life, as it is the same word in ancient Egyptian, and scarabs were many times used as seals to bind spells; otherwise this was made symbolically by the hands of the magician. Ancient Egyptians related every thought to what happened in nature, the scarab represented the solar cycle, as it appeared every morning pushing its dung ball (a connotation with the sun disc) and continued to do so all day, reappearing again the next day.

The papyri-amulet were written in narrow bands of papyrus of six cm[496] up to a meter length and used as portable amulets; there is in Turin the largest specimen measuring 104x83 cm and with 120 lines.;[497] they had a type of decree-blessing from some gods, protecting the individual from diseases, evil eye and misfortunes of all types,[498] explicitly written in the roll. Many royal documents were written in papyrus (roll). Rolled and kept in a skin, wood or gold box, they were used around the neck or the arm.[499]

In Coptic examples, the *Michigan Papyrus* 593, the items 25 and 26 mention the manufacture of papyri-amulet containing the spell text.[500]

After this habit disappeared in Egypt, it continued in Nubia and it is still used today in certain parts of Oriental Africa. There are two specimens in the Louvre Museum and other in the Berlin Museum.

The stelae of Horus or *cippus* were another type of apotropaic amulet against evil animals such as snakes and scorpions, very popular in later periods of Egyptian history.[501]

The main figure was the Horus child in his human form, naked, bearing the side lock of youth with his feet standing on crocodiles as shown in numerous stelae in Museums such as the British Museum, the Metternich Stela at the Metropolitan Museum of New York and the Museum of Budapest. The power of the stela was revealed after being rinsed through water whilst reciting magical formulae for protection. The power inscribed in the stela's hieroglyphs passed on to the water and that water was drunk after or used in a bath for the querent to grant him/her the desired protection.[502] The example which is the most complex, the stela of Metternich, at the Metropolitan Museum of New York shows texts with magical and religious detail and spells against scorpion bites and the treatment from the action of its' venom.[503]

2.4. Human substances used as ingredients

The preparation and mixture of prescriptions were part of the magician's manual ritual. The use of ingredients themselves were not as effective as the words recited whilst it was being made. There are references to amulets made of herbs and animal remains all wrapped in linen[504] but none survived until today.

Therefore the amulet was composed of a group of objects or substances and not just by a single piece.[505] The body areas most commonly used to wear amulets were the neck, the belly and the stomach.[506]

Human substances were common ingredients in spells; the excrements[507] or faeces (represented by the hieroglyphic character F52 from Gardiner), were offered to demons as they were considered filthy; these would be their food, the good food was offered to the gods.[508]

In the Coffin Texts there are three types of substances mentioned that the deceased must avoid; excrement or faeces, *hes,* urine, *ueseshet, wsšt*[509] and finally, *http-k'*, "the satisfaction of the *ka*", as a synonym of "filth".[510] In Text 193, it is said "O filth, I will not eat you with my mouth"; in Text 194 a recitation is made not to ingest faeces and a suggestion for the deceased to avoid to eat the dust from the ground; other texts suggest the deceased to avoid putrefact substances and debris. In Text 190 the alternative is given to the deceased; it suggests that the deceased has the knowledge to eat white emmer and drink water issuing from springs. Other food suggested elsewhere is: bread, red emmer, cakes, white emmer beer, cucumbers, grapes, and figs.[511]

The majority of references to these substances in the Coffin Texts are made to faeces; fewer explicit references are made to drinking urine.[512] And even less references to the "satisfaction of the *ka*"; maybe a lesser function. These sequences refer frequently to the consumption of food in opposition to the consumption of faeces and those are indicative of instructions for nutrition and distancing for the deceased.[513] These references to consume faeces and to drink urine in the Coffin Texts have their positioning around the legs and feet of the deceased inside the sarcophagus.[514]

At least nineteen types of excrements,

---

[496] Examples at the British Museum EA 10321, EA 10083 in Pinch, 1994: 36-37.
[497] Kakosy, Roccati, 1999: 118-119.
[498] Pinch, 1994: 142-143.
[499] Pinch, 1994: 117.
[500] Meyer, Smith, 1994: 300, 307.
[501] Pinch, 1994: 110, 143-144; Nagy, 1999: 90.
[502] Nagy, 1999: 91.
[503] Allen, 2005: 49-63.

[504] Pinch, 1994: 108.
[505] Pinch, 1994: 108.
[506] Pinch, 1994: 111-112.
[507] Pinch, 1994: 134.
[508] Borghouts, 1978: 6, 18.
[509] Faulkner, 2006: 69.
[510] Robinson, 2007: 148.
[511] Robinson, 2007: 150.
[512] Robinson, 2007: 154.
[513] Robinson, 2007: 155.
[514] Robinson, 2007: 156.

faeces, *hes* ⸝⸝⸝ *ḥs*,[515]

urine, *ueseshet* ⸝⸝⸝ *wsšt*,[516]

purge, *ueha* ⸝⸝⸝ *wḥȝ*,

vomit, *khaa* ⸝⸝⸝ *ḳȝ'*; are described as being used in ingredients for treatments.

The blood[517] was also used as ingredient, the menstrual blood considered repulsive and therefore used as bearer of evil things. The blood circulation was not understood as such; blood was another substance and its' circulation

part of the rest circulating in channels, the *metu* .

The saliva (spit, as it was connotated with the act of

spitting *peseg*, ⸝⸝⸝ *psg*,[518] was used as protection.

Tears, *remedj*, ⸝⸝⸝ *rmṯ*, were also much used in magic-inductive prescriptions. Ancient Egyptians considered that the annual flood came from the tears of Isis crying for her dead husband, killed by Seth, their brother.

Urine, *ueseshet*, had two implications; protector and repellent. The urine of pregnant women was considered a bearer of life. There is a story of an Egyptian prince who, to cure blindness, used urine from a woman who had never cheated on her husband, for a long period of time.[519]

---

[515] Faulkner, 2006: 177.
[516] Faulkner, 2006: 69.
[517] Pinch, 1994: 134.
[518] Faulkner, 2006: 95.
[519] Herodotus, 2003: 137.

Chapter 3
Types of diseases

There were several prescriptions for the same illness; according to the age and sex of the patient, of a quick or more slow action and manufactured according to the season of the year (For example, for ophthalmological diseases, the *Ebers Papyrus* 388 refers to the preparation of a prescription being made between the third to the fourth month of Winter)[520] as it was influenced by sun exposure to produce the desired effect.

An adult could take pills or a drinkable solution, a crushed medicine, but a baby could only have the medicine dissolved in the mother's milk. The weight and height of the person were also important to the manufacture of the prescription.

3.1. Parasitical

In the Egyptian concept the body belongs to Ra and each part has its own protector; the whole body has a network of channels, *metu*; respiratory tract, tear duct, glandular channels of all types, sperm channel and ligaments as well as substances flowing in those: blood, *senef*[521]

snfw; urine, *ueseshet, wsš*. These *metu* were identified with the Nile channels[522] and it was thought that air came through the nose and ears. The *metu* converge at the anus and if obstructed, give origin to diseases.

According to Lefebvre,[523] *metu*:

Designates, by principle the fibrous tissue that we call ligaments and the contractible tissue we call muscles. Another meaning for *met*, the most frequent, is vessel, in the sense that ancient Egyptians understood.
According to Jonckheere:[524]

- *met* is an anatomical word that, for ancient Egyptians, refers either to channel, as tendon or muscle and yet another type of formation, a type of channel in general.
Bardinet[525] says that:
- The word *metu* refers to several channels in the body. These are not solid strings; they are only there to ensure the current (movement as in machines). Through them, the nutritive elements, different fluids and the breath of life travel.
There were also evil ingredients and substances, the *wekhedw*, the transmitting agents of pain and disease. Being so, ancient Egyptians thought that the anus was the

centre of the majority of treatments. The cure of all diseases consisted in rest, a proper diet and the administration of medicine with frequent purges. We can draw conclusions on the way of life in ancient Egypt, as there were no significant changes until then, given the prevalence of the climate, food habits and endogenous diseases. The Egyptians thought that all men were healthy and that all disease has its' causes; visible or occult; internal or external:

External: (exogenous), eating too much, drinking too much, transmitted by air and insects.
Internal: (endogenous), the *wekhedw* originated by a putrid process in the intestines that circulates within the rest of the body.

Its removal was therefore vital, that is why they performed frequent purges to cleanse the body of unwanted substances. The causes could be food poisoning; and the expression used as disease, the *aaa*, an infectious disease circulating inside the body; with large probabilities of having cancerous characteristics.

Some translations from the *Ebers Papyrus* make repeated reference to the difficulty in diagnosing diseases with the name *aaa*. Attempts to interpret this were, until now, inconclusve. The paragraph 62 from the *Ebers Papyrus* relates *aaa* to a specific parasite that led some contemporary scholars to identify it as hematuria.[526] But other medical papyri give it a supernatural origin, a kind of punishment from the gods which enters the human body and circulates in it, causing unrest. The *aaa* is mentioned fifty times, in four papyri; (28 in the *Ebers Papyrus*, twelve in the *Berlin Papyrus*, nine in the *Hearst Papyrus*, and once in the *London Papyrus*.[527]

Another possibility for *aaa* is that it is the endemic schistosomiasis (bilhiarziosis) but it would not be possible for ancient Egyptians to observe the parasite in order that they could identify it. The concept of *aaa* can also be interpreted as semen or venom. In medical papyri there are many references to worms being responsible for occupying and destroying the body. Regarding possible causes for disease, according to ancient Egyptians, from the sources available, these would be *les agents provocateurs*, or pathogenic circulating elements: the *aaa*, *wekhedw* [528]and other creations

---

[520] Bardinet, 1995: 309.
[521] Nunn, 1996: 225.
[522] Cuenca-Estrella, 2004: 62.
[523] Lefebvre, 1952: 7.
[524] Jonckheere, 1947: 17-9.
[525] Bardinet, 1995: 64-65.

[526] An abnormal presence of blood in urine.
[527] David, 2000, 32, 1: 133-135.

[528] Steuer, 1948. It is curious that Gardiner interprets the sign Aa2, as pustule or gland in his *Egyptian Grammar; Being an Introduction to the Study of Hieroglyph*, which makes us think of a cyst or tumour. According to Steuer, ancient Egyptians wrongly mistake pus from a wound or diagnosed pathology, showing decomposing tissue at the

from Seth, the incarnation of evil and disorder. The blood, *senef*, generally considered as beneficial but also quoted in some medical texts as a substance that corrodes and a pathogenic element. This blood 'that eats',[529] according to texts, can block the passage of the breath of life.

The *aaa*, a body emanation of divine essence, can also be an intestinal parasite. It can become *wekhedw* when decomposing. A passage in the *Ebers Papyrus* indicates that its origin is in the body; a kind of body secretion or fluid issued by gods or demons, able to originate parasites. In the same passage the *aaa* is grease.[530] The *wekhedw* are evil elements related to decomposed matter. They come from faecal substances and their presence is a synonym of aging and death.

Both in the *Ebers Papyrus* and the *Hearst Papyrus* and *Berlin Papyrus* 3038, the *wekhedw* gather two principles, one non-medical (the demonic ability that enters the body from its' exterior and another, from the faecal matter that enters blood and infects it).[531] These would be substances animated by a pathogenic breath opposing all processes of cicatrisation.[532] And there is also the *wehaw*, secretions or pus caused by the *wekhedw*. A passage in the *Ebers Papyrus* 103 states that *wekhedw* produce *wehaw* [hieroglyphs], a non-identified skin disease according to Nunn,[533] such as urticaria (hives), a skin eruption caused by an infection as shown by the determinative of pustule in the name.[534] The *setet*: some authors translated these as rheumatisms as they cause pain as they travel in the body channels, dead or alive. If they are killed by an ill-inspired doctor, they become even more terrible.[535] All these considerations, running around the mind of ancient Egyptians, would be conclusive of an analysis with scientific purpose although it had its quota of magic.

3.1.1. Plagues/Infestations

Many insects tormented ancient Egyptians: flies, mosquitoes and grasshoppers. At the least, they were just disturbing; at worst, they could lead to famine, even by praying to the gods, sometimes a plague could not be prevented. The cattle were also threatened and crops were invaded by a destroying scarab. Mosquitoes and parasites were devastating for the population, polluting the still

waters of channels and Nile lakes. The fresh oil from the *ben* plant or a network was considered effective as a repellent, because mosquitoes were very disturbing to sleep (even today...).

To fumigate a house with incense and myrrh was recommended but not accessible to all; with *kyphi*,[536] a compound of incense used in ancient Egypt for religious and medical purposes. The word is Greek; *kyphi* is the transcription from the Egyptian *kepet*.[537] The oldest reference dates from the Coffin Texts[538] a list of all the goods the king will enjoy in the afterlife. The *Harris Papyrus* I [539] has a record of a donation and delivery of plants and resins for its' manufacture in the temples of Ramesses III. The instructions for the preparation of *kyphi* and respective list of ingredients were found in the inscriptions of walls at the temples of Edfu and Dendera. Dioscorides also speaks of the preparation of *kyphi* in his *Materia Medica*, thought to be the first Greek description of these materials. Galen preserves a medical poem where he includes *kyphi,* translated from Damocrates, and referring to *mithridatium* or *mithridaticum*, a semi-mystical prescription with at least 65 ingredients, used as an antidote for poisonings. In *Isis and Osiris*, Plutarch[540] comments about Egyptian priests burning incense three times a day: incense (pure) at dawn, myrrh at noon, and *kyphi* at sunset.

He relates about *kyphi*'s ingredients, sixteen, "These are composed, not at random, but, while sacred writings are read to perfume holders as they stir the ingredients." Plutarch adds that the mixture was used as a potion. All *kyphi* prescriptions mention wine, honey and raisins. Other ingredients include cinnamon (*Cinnamomum zeylanicum*), cassia (*Cinnamomum cassia*),[541] aromatic rhizomes from cypress (*Cupressus sempervirens*), cedar, juniper berries, incense resins, myrrh, benzoin resin[542] and mastic gum (*Pistacia lentiscus*).[543] Even though, in Egyptian prescriptions there are still unknown ingredients. The result of this mixture was displayed in balls and burnt in hot coal to exhale its' perfume.[544]

The first record of a human death linked to an insect is a sting from a wasp inflicted on King Menes or Narmer the one who unified Upper and Lower Egypt.[545]

---

moment of embalming. Therefore this determinative is shown in both medical papyri and mummification descriptions. The sign Aa3 from

[hieroglyph]

Gardiner seems to be the evolution of the first; when a secretion of substances for the exterior of tissues is flowing, such as the case of fluids leaking in inflammations, infections and other trauma.

[529] Bardinet, 1995: 335 (*Ebers Papyrus* 592-602).
[530] Bardinet, 1995: 121.
[531] Steuer, 1948: 14.
[532] *Ebers Papyrus* 86.
[533] Nunn, 1996: 226.
[534] *Ebers Papyrus* 91-92; 138.
[535] *Ebers Papyrus* 51, 15-52, 7; 102 and 296; *Berlin Papyrus* 142-143.

[536] Manniche, 1989: 57-58; Loret, 1887.
[537] Pujol, 2004 http://www.Egyptlogia.com/content/view/513/45/1/2/
[538] Mercer, 1952.
[539] *Papyrus British Museum EA* 9999, the largest Papyrus found until today, with 1500 lines, found at Medinet Habu, and bought by Anthony Charles Harris in 1855; came to the British Museum collection in 1872.
[540] Plutarco, 2001.
[541] Cinnamon and cassia were also used in mummification, http://www.unlv.edu/Faculty/landau/herbsandspices.htm
[542] This resin, extracted mainly from *Styrax benzoides* and *Styrax benzoin*, is native to Asia. It would have been imported into Egypt. The tree bark is dried and then used in perfumes, incense and medicine.
[543] *Pistacia lentiscus*. Mastic or lentisc resin was found in residues inside Egyptian amphorae, in Serpico, 2003: 462-464,467.
[544] Manniche, 1989; Plutarco, 2001.
[545] Krombach, Kampe, Keller, Wright, 2004:1234.

It could have been a specimen of the fig-wasp (*Blastophagus psenes*). This species helps pollenate fig trees; it appears, spontaneously, or by introduction, in the majority of locations where fig trees are grown (*Ficus carica*).[546]

Koji Nakanishi[547] who lived in Egypt, worked with toxins from wasps, to synthesize compounds similar to the venom of a type of Egyptian wasp, making them thirty times stronger. Wasps live in holes in trees such as sycamores and they are vital to the development fruit bearing seeds.

Stings and animal bites, such as those from snakes, scorpions and some insects are referred to in the prescriptions from the *Brooklyn Papyri*; BM 9997, BM 10309, BM 10085, BM 10105[548])
Even singing birds could represent a plague although they were very useful as they ate insects, they also searched fruit trees to eat sprouts when they are not yet ripen. Therefore, ancient Egyptians had frequently displayed nets in the trees, stuck by sticks, so that, as birds flew lower and rested in tree branches, the sticks were removed, leaving the birds powerless and easily captured.

The best way to keep a house free of rodents was to clean it constantly and to have a cat. Rats carried several diseases, invading barns and ruining crops which were vital to the population. In some domestic houses we can see how the inhabitants tried to prevent rats from coming inside, for example, holes in walls are filled with rocks; rats were also prevented from entering homes using cats and iron sticks. The *Ebers Papyrus* mentions methods to prevent rodent plagues. Some seem very practical but others are purely magical. Cat's grease was also useful, it was unbearable for rats[549] and used to protect cereals from rats, burnt excrement from deer was also used.

House insects were killed by washing the house with natron or washing the walls with *bebit*, *bb-t*, mixed with crushed coal.[550] As insects are less active in lower temperature, barns were built generally underground.

The same natron, an onion bulb or a dried fish, *tilapia Nilotica* were put in front of the wall or ground hole to prevent snakes from coming out.[551]

Goose's grease was also effective against flies, eradicating them, and fish' eggs drove fleas away. These should be abundant as the *Ebers Papyrus* has two prescriptions against them.[552]

Ashes dispersed around cereals in the mill killed scarabs. The protection from beasts (feline) was effective if an acacia was planted.

Using the right spell enhances also protection...

Parasitical diseases vehicled by water - ingestion

Disease	Etiological agent
Ascaridiasis, a benign parasitosis caused by the nematode worm *Ascaris lumbricoides*, (transmission by ground dust is frequent)	*Ascaris lumbricoides* (helmint)
Dracunculosis (dracontiasis)	*Dracunculus medinensis* (nematode, Guinea worm)
Tricuriasis (tricocefaliasis transmission by ground dust is frequent)	*Trichuris trichiura* (nematode)

Parasitical diseases vehicled by water – direct contact

Schistosomiasis (bilhiarziosis) infection caused by water snail. The bacterium enters skin through blood stream causing anaemia, loss of appetite, and urinary infection. A possibility for the *aaa* disease, that Egyptians tried to cure with circumcision and the use of antimony. At the tomb of Ankhnmahor at Saqqara, vizier and priest of *ka*, from the VIth Dynasty c. 2200 BC, there is a depiction of ceremonial circumcision.[553]	*Schistosoma (mansoni, haematobium and japonicum* - trematode)
Pruride of swimmers	*Schistosoma* (from birds and rodents - trematode)

Diseases transmitted by vectors (reproducing in water)

Disease	Agent	Vector
Filariosis	*Wuchereria bancrofti* (helmint)	Mosquito (several species)
Trypanosomiasis	*Trypanosoma* (protozoary)	Fly (Tsé-Tsé Glossina)

The table shows examples of more frequent parasitical diseases in ancient Egypt, according to several medical articles and interpretations from translations made by Egyptologists on the several medical Papyri containing therapeutics for 'worm' diseases.[554] Comparison with present data confirms that these are still the more common infections in Egypt as in Africa and other

---

[546] Ramirez, 1070:680.
[547] New York Columbia University Department of Chemistry, "I can explain the principle behind a good science experiment in 15 seconds; the same with magic."
http://www.columbia.edu/cu/chemistry/groups/nakanishi/
[548] Leitz, 1999: 3-30, 85-92.
[549] Bardinet, 1995: 362 (*Ebers Papyrus* 847); Lisboa, 1978: 284; Ebeid, 1999: 353.
[550] Ebeid, 1999: 351 (*Ebers Papyrus*, 840).
[551] Bardinet, 1995: 361 (*Ebers Papyrus de*, 842).; Ebeid, 1999: 356; Koenig, 1979:108.

[552] Lisboa, 1978:284.
[553] Herodotus, 2003: 109; his ironic tone in describing this practice, reflects his opinion on aesthetics, not taken into account by priests when circumcising, distinguishing between daily activities of Egyptians as "filthy" comparing to Greek's. This analogy, to Herodotus, shows a paradox in the concern with circumcision as a method for prophylactic medicine.
[554] The woman from Punt at the temple of Hatshepsut shows large legs, probably swollen from the accumulation of lymph, obstructed by an infection caused by as insect sting.

developing countries with identical climate conditions as some areas in India and South Asia. [555]

Poliomyelitis

The equine foot would have been documented maybe for the first time in history, in ancient Egypt.[556]

It is a viral infection of the cells in the spinal cord[557] which is only identified in those who survive the disease. Some examples from ancient Egypt: a shortening of the left leg in a mummy from Deshasha[558] was interpreted as being poliomyelitis. Siptah's twisted foot[559] as well as the deformities in the mummy of Khnumunakht from the XIIth Dynasty are also probably cases of poliomyelitis.[560] A funerary stela from the XVIIIth or XIXth Dynasty shows the doorman Roma with a shortened leg with an equine deformity in his foot (*talipes equinovorus*), *deneb*[561] in ancient Egyptian. Some think today that it is poliomyelitis contracted in childhood before the whole human skeleton is completed, but the foot deformity could be a compensation of the shortened leg of Roma.[562]

3.2. Dermatological

Ancient Egyptians were, throughout all their lives, concerned with beauty and youth and this is shown by the existence of special cosmetic care with medicinal properties. Dying hair, using unguents to make a body firm, perfumes dripping down heads eliminating parasites and evil smells, had an antiseptic property, all these had one aim, to combat aging. There are at least three sources describing these concerns; the *Ebers Papyrus*; the *Edwin Smith Papyrus*; the *Hearst Papyrus*, where it lists how to remove grey hair; (*Ebers Papyrus* 451, 452, 459 to 461).

To prevent the loss of pigment in hair; (*Ebers* 453 to 458, 462, 463; *Hearst* 147 to 149); to make hair grow (baldness was a large concern,[563] as superior social status given to priests that shaved all hair was not the same as being bald, for an Egyptian hair loss represented a loss in vitality (*Ebers* 464 to 467, 468 for women, 469 to 473; *Hearst* 144 to 146), but also the removal of hair was done to enhance the body beauty (*Ebers* 476, 774; *Hearst* 155, 156). To look younger (face - *Ebers* 716 to 721), for skin in general (*Ebers* 714 and *Hearst* 153 and *Smith* column 21, lines 3-6; *Ebers* 715 and *Hearst* 154 and *Smith* column 21, lines 6-8; *Smith* column 21, line 9 to column 22, line 10).

The evil smells also had their own prescriptions; (*Ebers* 708 to 711; *Hearst* 31, 32 and 150, 151).

Some weeds from the Nile banks treated skin-*inm* diseases, such as vitiligo (*vitiligo lymphoma*),[564] psoriasis and others. The lesions from vitiligo were treated with extract of *Ammi majus L.* (bishop's weed), followed by sun exposure as mentioned in the *Ebers Papyrus*.

The oedema, a chronic disease in which water is retained between skin tissues, was described with a hieroglyph that meant "water below the skin", 〰〰 ΥΥ 〰〰, *mui, nwi*; described in case 4 from the *Edwin Smith Papyrus*[565] and this hieroglyph was similar to the Nile annual flood.

Psoriasis

This disease was treated in ancient Egypt using phyto-photodermatitis, which is a photosensitive dermic reaction induced by exposure to certain plants, with subsequent solar exposure. The two agents are necessary to the efficacy of the treatment. Plants with these characteristics are: celery (*Apium graveolens*), turnip (*Brassica campestris*), fennel (*Foeniculum vulgare*), tarragon (*Artemisia dracunculus*), anis (*Pimpinela anisum*), marine salt, lime (*Citrus aurantiifolia*), lemon (*Citrus limon*), rue (*Ruta graveolens*), fig (*Ficus carica*), mustard (*Brassica alba*), chrysanthemum and bergamot (*Monarda didyma*). In the records of ancient Egypt, garlic and aloe vera are also mentioned[566] mixed with other ingredients as cucumber and wine.

The psoralenes, also called furocumarins, are photosensitive agents found in these plants. These were known in ancient Egypt.[567] Psoralenes can be taken orally or applied directly on skin. They allow a minimal dose of UVA rays to be used. When combined with UVA exposure they are efficient in eradicating psoriasis. The reason is still unknown but it will surely have to be with cellular renewal which happens with combined exposure to the two agents and the response of our immune system.

Haircare

Baldness represented one of the largest concerns of Egyptian society as hair was considered both an aphrodisiac and a sign of youth. There were prescriptions to dye hair when it lost its pigmentation and also to grow more hair. This does not invalidate the ritual of total depilation that many Egyptians were submitted to,[568] even in the military[569] as sign of a social status.

Men were generally shaven and, during the Middle Kingdom and the New Kingdom shaving was done using

---

[555] Information taken from: http://www.saudepublica.web.pt/06-SaudeAmbiental/061-Aguas/AbastecimAgua_texto.htm, notes from medical lectures at Lisboa and medical reports studied at the Wellcome Institute in London.

[556] Newsom, 2005:14.

[557] Ebeid, 1999: 401.

[558] Or Dishasha, an Old Kingdom location with a cemetery c.130 km south of Cairo where Flinders Petrie excavated some tombs in 1898: University College of London:
http://www.digitalegypt.ucl.ac.uk/deshasheh/index.html

[559] Ebeid, 1999: 403; Fleming, Fishman, O'Connor, Silverman, 1980:85.

[560] Cockburn, 1998:43.

[561] Ebeid, 1999: 399.

[562] Nunn, 1996:77.

[563] Ebeid, 1999: 289.

[564] A pathology characterized by depigmentation of skin and hair which results in the appearance of light spots.

[565] Bardinet, 1995:496; Faulkner, 2006:105.

[566] Manniche, 1989: 70-72.

[567] Oliveira, 2005: vii.

[568] Ebeid, 1999: 351.

[569] Ebeid, 1999: 348.

copper and bronze blades, metals known for producing sharp edges, therefore many men trusted professional barbers. For the depilation of the body they used a mixture of crushed bird bones, oil, sycamore juice and gum, heated and applied onto skin. After cooling down, this hardened shell was removed, presumably removing hair. Scissors also were used:[570] *tj'ait-iret*, to remove unwanted hair. Wigs were used by men and women and they were made of human hair, and later from palm fibres that were curled.

3.3. Diabetes

The relationship between diabetes and kidneys would have been suggested for the first time by Aretaeus of Cappadocia. The first reference to *diabetes mellitus* is given to the *Ebers Papyrus*[571] that mentions prescriptions for treatment of excessive urine, (poliuria).[572] These prescriptions had a function: "to eliminate urine that is too much". The following prescription was prescribed for the treatment of poliuria: water from the lake where birds drink, wild berries, fibres from plant *asit*, fresh milk and bush from pigs soaked in beer, cucumber flowers, and unripened dates.

3.4. Tuberculosis

Man would have contracted this disease from bovines and the disease changed gradually in humans; this statement came from the fact that there is no trace of this disease in the pre-dynastic period, when there was no domestication of bovines. Andreas G. Nerlich[573] analyzed the DNA from 26 Theban mummies from the New Kingdom and Greco-Roman period; six of those had been infected with a human type of tuberculosis. He thinks that up to 50% of the Egyptian population could have been affected by tuberculosis. It is a viral infection in the intestines that can attack bone marrow and cause irreversible paralysis, generally in legs. Transmitted by faecal contamination in food and water, it is an asymptomatic disease; starting with fever, migraines and heat in the throat and has no treatment.

There is a documented case of an Egyptian mummy of an infant with tuberculosis found in the tomb of Nebuenenef (TT 157) that shows that this disease did not discriminate regarding age; the child would have contracted tuberculosis by close contact with an infected elderly person.[574] In modern immunological techniques it is possible to extract the bacteria from bone for identification and establish if it is of bovine origin or human. Tuberculosis of the vertebral column was found in Egyptian mummies from c. 3000 BC, the first existing record about this disease was the one from Hippocrates in

450. Later on, Sir Percival Pott,[575] in 1779, was the first author to make a detailed description of the disease; the word tuberculosis faded in 1839. It is a chronic infectious disease, endemic, caused by *Mycobacterium tuberculosis*, described by Robert Koch in 1882. It can also be caused in other ways, from *Mycobacterium* (*M. bovis*, *M. kansasin*, *M. fortuitum*, *M. martinum*, *M. intracellulase*).[576]

Ruffer[577] refers the presence of tuberculosis in the vertebral column of Nesiparehan, priest of Amun from the XXIth Dynasty. It shows the main characteristics of Pott's disease with a collapse of the thoracic vertebrae, producing kyphosis.[578] A known complication from Pott's disease is that the tuberculosis suppuration lowers down to the *psoas* muscle until the iliac fossa, producing a large *psoas* abscess.[579] Ruffer's report[580] refers to the best case of spinal tuberculosis in ancient Egypt.

All possible cases were examined from the pre-dynastic period to the XXIth Dynasty, by Morse, Brockwell, and Ucko[581] and by Buikstra, Baker, and Cook[582] in 1993. They have included *specimens* from Petrie and Quibell's Naqada in 1895 as well as nine Nubian specimens from the Royal College of Surgeons of England. Both teams had little doubt that tuberculosis was the pathological cause in most of them, but not all cases. In some cases it was not possible to exclude the compression of fractures, osteomyelitis, and bone cysts as causes of death.[583]

A representation of a hunchback was found on pre-dynastic ceramics in Aswan[584] representing a human with an angular kyphosis in the thoracic column, bended over an adobe construction. Another item indicating a vertebral deformity is a small representation of a human with arms folded at the elbows. It has a protrusion of the back and chest.[585]

The last example is a wooden statue at the Brussels Museum.[586]

It was bought in the auction from the Amherst collection at London in 1921 and it is only a naked torso and a head with a pointed beard. It does not show any of the upper limbs and from the lower limbs only a right thigh is present. It has a prominent thorax and an accentuated

---

[570] Ebeid, 1999: 128 (scissors belong to the group of instruments at the Cairo Egyptian Museum as stated by Ebeid).
[571] Abdelgadir, 2006: 11.
[572] Nunn: 1996: 91.
[573] Zink, 2001:.355-366.
[574] Zimmerman, 1979: 604-608.

[575] Pott, 1779.
[576] http://www.rbo.org.br/materia.asp?mt=1320&idIdioma=1
[577] Ruffer, 1910; Ebeid, 1999:146.
[578] Kyphosis, best known as hunchback, is defined as an abnormal increase of the anterior concavity of the vertebral column, the most important causes being bad posture and insufficient physical conditioning.
[579] Nunn, 2002.
[580] Ruffer, 1910.
[581] Morse, D., Brothwell, D. R., Ucko, P. J., *Tuberculosis in Ancient Egypt*, *American Review of Respiratory Disease* 90, 1964: 524-41.
[582] Buikstra, Baker, Cook, 1993.
[583] Nunn, 1996:73.
[584] Schrumph-Pierron, 1933
[585] Morse 1967: 261.
[586] Cuenca-Estrella e Barba, 2004: 42; Ebeid, 1999:145.

hunchback. From the paleopathological point of view this person would have suffered vertebral tuberculosis[587] in childhood which left permanent sequels.

Another suggestive specimen, from the XVIIIth Dynasty, which is at the World Museum of Liverpool, M3519, it is a wooden statuette of a female servant with visible angular kyphosis, probably caused by poor posture when carrying jars.[588] Another example from the Middle Kingdom, in a tomb painting from Beni Hasan shows a gardener with an angular kyphosis in the cervical-thoracic column.[589]

Pettigrew observed traces of tuberculosis in the lungs of Petmautiomes from which she has probably died.[590]

3.5. Leprosy (*Mycobacterium leprae*)

The cases of leprosy in ancient Egypt cannot be confirmed before the Greco-Roman period, until the discovery of the mummy of Irtisenu,[591] the *Ebers Papyrus* mentions what seems to be this infectious disease in the lungs in ns. 874 and 877.[592] In 1980 it was found in four skeletons from the Ptolemaic period. It is thought that this disease would have arrived in Egypt only with the armies of Alexander.[593]

3.6. Achondroplasia (Dwarfism)

Dwarfs, *nemu*, *nmw*,[594] are very much represented in ancient Egyptian art, (an example, Seneb, Chief of the manufacturers of cloths at the royal palace, is represented in his tomb with his family), as they had great social importance in ancient Egypt.[595] Veronique Dasen[596] indicates having studied more than a thousand representations of dwarfism in ancient Egypt. The majority are usually not very tall, with a head and torso of normal size and shorter limbs. The statue of Seneb is the classic example as it indicates that these people showed their acceptance in society very openly.

Another example quoted by Ruffer[597] includes a statuette from the Vth Dynasty, of Khnumhotep from Saqqara, the pre-dynastic drawing of the dwarf Zer from Abydos, and a drawing from the Vth Dynasty of a dwarf at the tomb of Deshasha. Because being physically handicapped in ancient Egypt showed sign of divinity, to be marked as someone special, or to have gifts that others do not have; many dwarfs and people with physical deformities, either genetic, congenital or resulting from diseases in childhood or from trauma (such as infections from tetanus),[598] could be prized by kings and obtain high status in society.

In the *Instructions of Amenemope* (BM 10474), acquired for the British Museum by Wallis Budge in his Egyptian expedition of 1887-88;[599] a text dealing with professions, where a high status employee gives advice to his son so that he follows the path of Truth, it is said in Chapter 25: "Do not laugh at a blind man. Nor tease a dwarf. Nor cause hardship for the lame. "[600] This text is distributed in several parts in various Museums: Turin, Italy, Pushkin Museum in Moscow, the Louvre, an Ostracon in Cairo and a fragment at Stockholm. Dated from the New Kingdom,[601] its' theme is much older. The largest part is in a manuscript, almost complete and it is thought to have been written just before the kingdom of Amenhotep III.

3. 7. Vascular diseases

Calcification of the aorta was discovered in two Egyptian mummies in 1852 and there are descriptions of temporal arteries with calculi in the mummy of Ramesses II and in Merenptahs' aorta, extreme calcareous degeneration with formations of plaques which looked just like bone were discovered. Ruffer, in his article about arterial lesions comments on the extreme mutilation caused during the process of embalming which, sometimes, just left the arteries of the arms and legs for examination, all the rest being pulled out by hand.[602]

Atherosclerosis

An example of atherosclerosis is reported by Moodie in an adult female mummy from the pre-dynastic period.[603] This disease, which appears to have been very prevalent in ancient Egypt[604] is present in the VIth Dynasty, c. 2345-2333 BC, as it is shown in the tomb of Teti at Saqqara, where two images make the distinction between death and fainting: the left hand in the head for death and the right hand in the head for fainting.[605]

In the torso of an adult male mummy of between 40 to 60 years of age, found in the tomb 93.11 at Dra Abu el-Naga, near Thebes[606] coronary atherosclerosis and miocardic fibrosis was detected in his heart. It is a genetic disease. Ruffer analyzed several arteries: aortas, carotid and iliac, with calcifications "decalcifying them" in a solution of alcohol at 98% and nitric acid at 2%.[607]

[587] http://www.globalegyptianMuseumm.org/record.aspx?id=885
[588] Reeves, 1992: 40.
[589] Cuenca-Estrella e Barba, 2004: 42. Tomb of Ipuy, XIXth Dynasty.
[590] Pettigrew, 1838:13.
[591] Ebeid, 1999:56
[592] Bardinet, 1995: 371-373.
[593] Ebeid, 1999:214-215.
[594] Dasen, 1988:258.
[595] Sullivan, 2001:262.
[596] Dasen, 1988:254.
[597] Ruffer, 1921: 48.

[598] Miller, 1997:758.
[599] Budge, 1920, 1:337.
[600] Lichtheim, 1997:121.
[601] XXII Dynasty, Budge, 1922: 431-432.
[602] Ruffer, 1921: fig.24.
[603] Moodie, 1931:20, 22.
[604] Moodie, 1931:26.
[605] Britto, Herrera, 2005:3.
[606] Nerlich, Wiest, Tubel, 1997:83. Deutsches Archaeologisches Institut in Cairo http://www.dainst.org/index_55_en.html
[607] Ruffer, 1921:13.

3. 8. Ophthalmological

Ophthalmological diseases in ancient Egypt included poor sight, strabismus, cataracts, conjunctivitis and trachoma. In order to reduce the aggressive effect of sunlight ancient Egyptians painted the area around the eyes with malachite, a green copper mineral, extracted from Sinai and oriental desert mines; also *mesdemet* or galena consisted of a cosmetic powder which protected the eyes from sand and wind and also from insect plagues.

Night blindness was cured using cooked and crushed ox liver[608] which is known to be very rich in vitamin A. Other diseases, cataracts and plaques that form and cause the loss of the eye's lenses transparency, the retina, as it was called in Latin, in analogy to a fluid flowing from the brain to the eyes... The Egyptians called it "the rising of the water",[609] reporting the same false conclusion that Romans did centuries later. The treatment was made with a mixture of turtle brain and honey. The first surgery was done at Alexandria during the Ptolemaic period (323 BC to 30 BC).

In the Coffin Texts n. 157 there is a reference to what seems to be the first eye examination which associated the pig with the loss of eyesight.[610] Could this be the reason for the prohibition of eating pork in Egypt?

Ebers Papyrus and ophthalmology

The *Ebers Papyrus* is dated by a passage in the verso as being from year 9 from the kingdom of Amenhotep I (c. 1534 BC). A large step in ophthalmology can be seen in this Papyrus, where a whole section is dedicated to eye diseases, more to treatments than clinical descriptions. It has also some spells and also evidence of scientific knowledge.

Inflammation of the eyelids[611] such as ciliary blepharitis[612] (inflammation of the eyelid margin) was present in ancient Egypt and was likely to be the condition that they referred to as "heat in the eye", *tj'u*.

A lump on the eyelid (*chalazion*)[613] or stye (*hordeolum*) infection of the sebaceous glands at the base of the eyelashes is a small abscess of the follicle of an eyelash. This is painless where usually there is an inflammation, acute and purulent of a sebaceous gland in the eyelash.

The *ectropion*;[614] in which the lower eyelid turns outwards, leaving the eye exposed and dry, is caused by lack of muscle tone in the eyelid; this also causes hypo or hyper secretion of tears and wiping them away only

aggravates the situation. It is a common disease in people over sixty years old, however, in Egypt this is an exception as it affects younger individuals. The *ectropion* may cause redness and hyper sensitivity to light and wind.

A lower eyelid turning inwards irritates the cornea,[615] *entropion* can cause blindness. *Trichiasis*,[616] an abnormal eyelid, defined by the direction of the eyelashes which turn inwards towards the eye, is another disease. It can be partial or total. The cause may be anatomical and it is more frequent in adults.

Other conditions: eye spots, *sehedju*,[617] or granulations, *chemosis* (conjunctive tissue filled with fluid; swollen eye or conjunctivitis), *pinguecula,* a benign yellow outgrowth, forming in the conjunctive tissue. These grow near the cornea. It is thought that *pingueculae* are caused by ultraviolet light and that they are more common in people spending too much time under the sun. It does not affect sight, but it can cause irritation if it grows too big. In rare cases the *pinguecula* may extend to the cornea, forming a *pterygium*.[618] These are abnormal outgrowths of conjunctive tissue common in people living in tropical climates or spending much time under the sun. They cause irritation, redness and tears.

The *pterygium*s are fed by miniscule hair. They may affect sight. As the *pterygium* is developing, it can alter the shape of the cornea, causing stigmatism. If the *pterygium* invades the central cornea, it can be surgically removed.

Other conditions: leucoma,[619] whitening and thickening of the cornea, either convex or protruding as a consequence of trauma or inflammation; iritis or inflammation of the iris; cataracts, inflammation of tear duct, and following inflammatory process causing inability of tear duct.

It is thought that the *Ebers Papyrus* was probably the product of priests (who were doctors too).
This follows the idea that part of the six volumes lost in Alexandria contained the "doctors' secrets".[620] There is no evidence of advancements in surgery; the closest mention in this papyrus is depilation, a much used practice judging by the frequency of forceps' drawings in New Kingdom reliefs. Herodotus reports that Cyrus of Persia asked Ahmes, c. 560 BC, king of the XXVIth Dynasty, a doctor for his eyes.[621]

The trachoma, *nehat*,[622] is an infectious disease very well known in antiquity, with references from ancient

---

[608] Nunn, 1996: 200; Ebeid, 1999: 155.
[609] Ebeid, 1999: 155.
[610] Ritner, 1997: 30.
[611] Nunn, 1996: 201.
[612] Ebeid, 1999: 154.
[613] Idem.
[614] Ebeid, 1999:154.

[615] Nunn, 1996: 201-202.
[616] Ebeid, 1999:154.
[617] Ebeid, 1999:156; Nunn, 1996: 202.
[618] Ebeid, 1999:154.
[619] Idem.
[620] Pinch, 1994: 133.
[621] Ebeid, 1999: 157.
[622] Nunn, 1996: 201.

Egypt.[623] It is discussed in the Ebers *Papyrus*. The bacterium *Chlamydia trachomatis* affects the eye spreading from the persons infected hands or clothing, or it can be passed on by insects, coming into contact with humans through the eyes or nose. As trachoma is transmitted by personal contact it usually occurs in small, closed communities. It does not lead to blindness straight away; but it works gradually.

This disease arrived in Europe with Napoleonic wars after French and English soldiers come back from Egypt. It was rapidly spread over the military camps as the hygiene conditions were poor.

At Deir el-Medina the workmen suffered from several diseases, blinding dust being the most frequent. In an ostracon from the XIXth Dynasty, a father writes to his son asking for treatment for his eyes; he, the father was a sketch artist, who wrote to his son, also a sketch artist, Pre [emhab?]:

"Do not turn your back on me; I am not well. Do not [stop] moaning me, as I am in the [darkness (?) since] myLord Amun [turned] his back on me. Can you bring some honey for my eyes, and also some ochre to make bricks other time, and black eye paint? [Quick!] Look! Am I not your father? Now, I am crippled; I search for my sight and it is not there. " [624]

Blindness was incapacitating and a sketch artist employed to create images and written hieroglyphic in tombs would be prevented from working properly. Descriptions of a mixture of honey, ochre black eye paint, which the father asks from his son, appear in medical papyri, as it should have been a common medicine then. Honey has antiseptic properties, and ochre, cools down the eyelids and reduces swellings. Many workers suffered from these eye concerns. "Cadmia[625] acts as a drying agent, cures wounds, stops bleedings, acts as detergent in webs and eye incrustations, removes eruptions, and produces, all good effects as led. Copper, when calcinated, is used for all purposes; including white spots and cicatrisation of eyes. Mixed with milk, it also cures eye wounds; and, for this specific purpose the people of Egypt manufactured a type of balm together with crushed stones. "[626]

3.9. Orthopaedic/Traumas

Starting by saying that there were diseases caused by trauma suffered in professional activities, as it is depicted in art, it is fare to say that the type of profession could determine the type of wounds or diseases accidentally, or maliciously caused.

The *Edwin Smith Papyrus* lists 48 cases of trauma, either caused in battle, violent arguments or handling heavy items. Osteo-articular deformities are shown in artistic depictions such as the one from the tomb of Ipuy at Deir el-Medina showing a dislocated shoulder;[627] the shepherd with a deformed knee at the mastaba of Ptahotep, Saqqara, Vth Dynasty; other deformities as an umbilical hernia, genital hypertrophy in fishermen and craftsman in the tomb of Mehu at Saqqara from the VIth Dynasty,[628] to name but a few.

Recent excavations at Deir el-Medina brought evidence of a brain 'surgery' undertaken on a workman who survived it another two years. Skeletons found at Tell Tabilla in June 2003 show symptoms of anaemia, osteoporosis, fractured and compressed vertebrae, and dental diseases and large abscesses. In robust male bodies cervical degenerations were found as well as an abnormal development of the arm muscle, which suggests carrying weights as the possible origin of muscular and bone problems. Traces of a distended hand were also found which suggests repetitive tasks using weights.[629]

From the analyzed cases we can conclude that, whoever lived into old age, (life expectancy was about 36 years,[630] between 35 and 40);[631] would suffer from arthritis (articulations were subjected to additional efforts in certain professions), atherosclerosis and dementia.[632] Rickets[633] was also diagnosed in an adult male mummy,[634] showing that this disease existed in ancient Egypt and it was not surely because they lacked vitamin D? Although there is no mention in the medical papyri, there is evidence that rickets existed in ancient Egypt.[635]

Migraines

To explain the origin of migraines in ancient Egypt and what the correspondent therapeutics was, there are several alternatives according to the source of the pain. In magical papyri migraines are caused by actions of demons and supernatural forces, in medical papyri its' cause is given to trauma and other pain felt in the body. Therefore the treatment could be magical, pharmacological or surgical.[636] In the *Ebers Papyrus* there are some prescriptions with treatments for migraine: 242-247; 250; 259. In the *Chester Beatty Papyrus* V, 4, 1-9, there is a reference to "head" in a prescription that includes magic and it is repeated seven times.[637]

[623] Medow, 2006
[624]http://www.mc.maricopa.edu/dept/d10/asb/anthro2003/legacy/ancient _lives/ostraca.html Universidade Mesa Community College, Arizona, USA
[625] From the Latin *cadmía*, the Greek *kadmeía*, a zinc carbonate extracted near Cadmo (Thebes); $ZnCO_3$
[626] Plínio, 2004, chapter 23.

[627] Ebeid, 1999:140; Nunn, 1996: 179; Filer, 1995: 33.
[628] Reeves, 1992: 34-35.
[629]Tell Tebilla Project http://www.deltasinai.com/delta-11.htm
[630] Lisboa, 1978:285.
[631] Fleming, Fishman, O'Connor, Silverman, 1980:74; Nunn, 1996:22.
[632] According to Zahi Hawass royal elites in ancient Egypt could reach 50 to 60 years of age.
[633] *Rachitis,* from the late Greek *rhachitis* «inflammation of the vertebral column» and the Greek *rhakhis* «spine».
[634] Moodie, 1931:22.
[635] Ebeid, 1999:396.
[636] Karenberg, Leitz, 2001: 911-916.
[637] Baptista, Meneghelli, Bordini, Speciali, 2003:53-54

Metabolic arthritis (gout)

There are records that Ptolemy II; Philadelphus suffered from gout.[638] This is a disease caused by a build up of uric acid deposited on the articular cartilage of joints, tendons and surrounding tissues causing inflammation and pain, the majority of cases were male showing symptoms in the feet, ankles, knees and elbows. The level of uric acid is increased to 85% of the cases.

This disease would have been treated by Erasistratus of Chios, 304BC-250BC,[639] when he prescribed a plaster for King Ptolemy's gout; the pain it gives is caused by excess food, excessive consumption of wine and a sedentary life. In coins of that period he is represented as a little over weight and this confirms his lifestyle. Nile water from the Alexandria area, saturated in mineral salts is an environmental factor to take into consideration but, a paradox is that water consumption is advised as it dilutes uric acid and helps in its expulsion from the body.[640]

Osteoporosis

This disease, (thinning bone, can be secondary to other disease) and osteopenia (recrudescence of bone mass above norm) was present in ancient Egypt populations.[641] Bones give some indications as Harris' lines (growth arrest lines) may be caused by bad nutrition, weakening bones and causing osteoporosis later on.[642]

In order to be visible in X rays these diseases have to surpass losses of more than 40%, in bone density, which is very difficult to find in archaeological material. The study of osteopenia via analysis of stable isotopes has been done in Egyptian mummies, although this technique requires destruction of bone samples. Therefore, the effects of alkaline phosphatase (an elevated enzyme when there is destruction of present bone) require the destruction of the organic material.

There is still no non-destructive method to apply in the investigation of epidemiology of osteoporosis and osteopenia in ancient Egypt. But dual energy X-ray absorptiometry (DXA technique), is used in present radiography to measure bone density and diagnose osteoporosis.[643]

Prosthetics

Prosthetic surgery must have existed[644] as prosthetics in ancient Egypt were generally used for aesthetic purposes; so that the person would not loose his/her complete physique, whether a toe, such as the one in British

Museum,[645] or a tooth replacing an incisor in the maxillary (jawbone)[646] or an arm such as the one from the mummy of Durham or a penis or a foot as kept at the Manchester Museum. There is another prosthetic of a wooden toe, from a woman aged between 50 and 60 years, after amputation of the large toe, in the Museum of Cairo.

A glass eye, missing the iris, would have belonged to a mummy much more probably than to a living person. Another example of a physical restoration was found in mummy 2343 from the Archaeological Museum of Naples where a radiographic exam showed wooden prosthetics in the place of feet. There are references to date these restorations with prosthetics to the Ptolemaic period,[647] which would place this mummy in the same period.

3.10. Oncological

All diagnosis up to date are controversial; what has been published since 1825 up to the present brings us to the conclusion that, as life expectancy was around 36 years old, the *aat* tumours would have affected essentially young people. From the analysis made, excluding bone tumours, it is thought that soft tissue tumours were essentially billiary[648] (given the high level of infection in the water snail), liver, nasopharynx and uterus. More rare tumours could have been breast and colo-rectal.[649]

In one study, around fifty cases of bone tumours in Egypt and Nubia were diagnosed as malignant,[650] and benign. Their classification amongst the cases reviewed in this study, made by an Italian team, has the following statistics:[651]

Osteosarcoma – 6; multiplex myeloma – 8; osteolytic metastatic carcinoma– 17; mixed metastatic carcinoma– 4; nasopharyngeal carcinoma – 7; others (male, osteolytic

---

[638] From the Latin *gutta*, literally gout.
[639] Erasistratus and Herophilus dissected bodies in Alexandria and were considered the fathers of neuroscience.
[640] Tunny, 2001: 119.
[641] Pesed referred in the table of doctors.
[642] Nunn 1996: 83.
[643] Haigh, 2000.
[644] Győry, 2006: 2.

[645] British Museumm EA 29996.
[646] Irish, 2004: 645.
[647] Guiffra, 2006: 274-278.
[648] There is record of an analysis done to a mummy of a priestess of Thebes's c. 1500 BC, at the Royal College of Surgeons Museum of London that showed a well preserved gall bladder with 30 calculi; unfortunately this mummy was destroyed in the Second World War bombings, as referred by Knut Haeger in *The Illustrated History of Surgery*. A more recent example of liver and gall bladder pathologies is Umm Kulthum, Arabic song diva, (May 4, 1904 –Feb 3, 1975), who became sick in the 1930 's; at the end of the summer of 1937 doctors advised her to have mineral water treatments. Next summer, Umm Kulthum spent a month in Vichy and came back to Egypt feeling better, although, according to her: «I am restricted by the limitations of a rigid diet that forbids the majority of food»; later on she died of nephritis, an inflammation in the kidneys caused by an infection.
[649] The author have described 72 cases of tumours found in ancient Egyptian material by several researchers in another work: Veiga, 2008, *Oncology and infectious diseases in ancient Egypt, The Ebers Papyrus' Treatise on Tumours 857-877 and the cases found in ancient Egyptian human material*, dissertation submitted to the University of Manchester for the degree of Master of Science in Biomedical and Forensic Studies for Egyptology
[650] 28 malignant in ancient Egypt: Gamba, Fornaciari, 2006:1.
[651] Giuffra, Ciranni, Fornaciari, 2007, 1-3.

in right maxillary), (female, ovarian bilateral cistoadenocarcinoma) – 2.

There is also a case exhibited at the Natural History Museum in London of a humerus demonstrating what might be diagnosed as a chondroblastic tumour. Other examples include benign tumours in skulls and, at Deir el-Medina, the case of a woman where a malignant tumour destroyed the facial skeleton. She may have lost her eyesight as a consequence of the neoplastic invasion of the orbit.[652]

A case found at Naga ed-Der, Upper Egypt, 235 kilometers north of Luxor, in tomb n. 217, which can be found today at the Lowie Museum of Anthropology, Berkeley, USA, shows a skull with extensive destruction. A large part of the face, with the exception of the orbits and the sphenoid region are destroyed, probably by a soft tissue tumour in the nasopharyngeal area. The eroded bone edges reveal osteolites of malignant nature and this indicates a probable carcinoma.[653]

Five cases of soft tissue tumour originating in the nasopharyngeal region [654] were detected in Egypt and Nubia which indicates that the incidence of this type of carcinoma in Africa (7.8%) is much more frequent than in the west. Four are Byzantine/Christian period cases (300-1400), and this may reveal an increase in the incidence of this type of carcinoma. Environmental conditions may favor this carcinoma as the Epstein-Barr virus thrives in Egypt.[655]

Some fatty acids are the promoters of viral infection and these are found in the plants *Euphorbiacea*,[656] typical of hot climates.

The inscriptions in the *Edwin Smith* and *Ebers Papyri* make distinction between benign and malignant tumours. The ones found at the surface of the skin were surgically removed (cysts). To treat tumours in the stomach and the uterus a mixture of barley, pigs' ears and other ingredients was made. It is also very probable that a multilocular cyst [657] found by Salama in the mandibular ramus of a 2,800 B.C. Egyptian mummy was a keratocyst. It was not associated with an impacted tooth and had greatly expanded the overlying cortices, causing a pathological fracture. This skull also contained a dentigerous cyst around the crown of an impacted

maxillary bicuspid, which may suggest Gorlin's syndrome or basal cell nevus syndrome.[658]

Strouhal has diagnosed 44 cases of bone neoplasms[659] eight were malignant. They include one observed by Granville in 1821 and diagnosed as an ovarian carcinoma from Irtusenu (mummy at the British Museum), an incorrect diagnosis as it was analyzed by Tapp in 1994 and the lesion is benign.[660]

In another study the remains of 905 individuals were analyzed[661] from three different areas of ancient Egypt[662] and 39 neoplasms were detected.

3.11. Dentists, teeth and dentistry

Teeth had several names, maybe because they had different physiology and Egyptians had already a notion on their differences, *ibeh*, ⟨𓄹⟩ *ibḥ* and *nehedjet*, ⟨𓄺⟩ *nḥdt*,[663] (the latter maybe referring to molars, according to Lefebvre[664]); are the hardest and more indestructible human tissues.[665] The determinative used is a fang, probably from an elephant, in the Egyptian way of representing human body parts through their animal counterpart.

In ancient Egypt, the most common dental problems were caries and abrasion (wear caused by chewing hard food).[666] With time, the enamel and dentine become so worn that the pulp is exposed. The result is a painful chronic infection. Periodontal disease,[667] very common in ancient Egypt, has many examples in mummies.[668]

A female mummy found next to the pyramid of Pepi I at Saqqara exhibits some lesions associated to her profession: the treatment of leather strings. The abnormalities found in the spaces between the superior incisors are coin-shaped and the dentine is showing; this suggests that it was a much repeated routine.[669]

---

[652] Tumours are called de neoplasias as they are new (neo) formations, between benign and malignant, and those are called cancers too; Campillo, 2001: 150.

[653] Strouhal, 1978: 290-302.

[654] The word cancer has its origin in Hippocrates, who used the Greek words *karkinos* (crab) and *karcinoma* to describe tumours as they were similar in shape.

[655] Epstein-Barr, virus *Lymphocryptovirus*, human virus of herpes 4, causing mononucleosis and associated to Burkitt's lymphoma and nasopharynx carcinoma, identified in 1964.

[656] *Ricinus communis* (ricin oil), part of the waste 'mash' when castor oil is manufactured.

[657] Hilmy, 1951; 90:17-18.

[658] Professor Gorlin suggested that it might best be called the nevoid basal cell carcinoma syndrome, although 10% of adults do not develop basal cell carcinomas (BCCs),
http://www.gorlingroup.co.uk/syndrome.htm, it has a dermatological appearance but after death it is diagnosed by the associated skeletal abnormalities, (Ebeid 1999: 103). This syndrome is characterized by multiple cutaneous nodules not exposed to the sun that tend to become malignant with age (basal cell nerves); multiple odontogenic keratocysts.

[659] Spigelman, Bentley, 1997:107.

[660] Spigelman, Bentley, 1997:107.

[661] Nerlich, Rohrbach, Bachmeier, Zink, 2006, 197-202.

[662] Abydos, Western Thebes TT196 and the third from Western Thebes also with no designation of the tomb: Nerlich, Rohrbach, Bachmeier, Zink, 2006, 198.

[663] Nunn, 1996:50.

[664] Lefebvre, 1956:60.

[665] Prof. Eugénia Cunha in a session of Forensic Anthropology at the Instituto de Medicina Legal de Lisboa, February 2007.

[666] Schwarz, 1979:37.

[667] From the Greek *pyórrhoia*, suppuration; a chronic pathology of gums characterized by progressive destruction of tissue.

[668] Moodie, 1931:25.

[669] Janot, 2003:37-39.

A mummified head, female and estimated to have lived more than 60 years of age, was found in tomb K95 at Dra Abu el-Naga, necropolis of Thebes and was identified as having the *corynebacterium* bacterium present in a dental abscess. From the remains of around forty individuals found in the same tomb it cannot be said that the bacterium was originated in this body and then contaminated another body. It was through DNA analysis that the bacterium could be identified but its type is not possible to get. But the reference in magical texts of a childs disease, *baa*, ⌐⌐⌐⌐⌐, *b''* may help in the characterization (*Berlin Papyrus 3027*). A myth described in *Papyrus Ramesseum III*, B, 23-24 reports Horus' experience recovering from *baa*.[670]

Periodontal disease (gingivitis) was really a problem. Calculus deposits (tartar) in teeth were frequent; the result is advanced loss of bone tissue, loose teeth, infection and subsequent loss of teeth. In dental caries the rapid wear creates cavities. A reason for this may be the absence of refined carbohydrates in diet. Some restorations can be observed in mummified Egyptian bodies.

In a case lacking three teeth, three substitute teeth were put in place with a gold wire.[671] Their diet, bread made with thick flour, which included sand would be the main cause of abrasion in teeth.[672] Dentists are known in Egypt since the Old Kingdom.[673] The first reference to the title of dentist was given to Hesire, c. 2650 BC; Herodotus mentions fifty names with the title of dentist. But Warren R. Dawson disagrees, saying that it is less likely that there were distinct medical professions before the Ptolemaic period.[674] Ruffer also says that his studies have not confirmed that there were dentist surgeons in ancient Egypt as mummies showed teeth that could have been treated or extracted to relieve pain...[675]

There were two classes of dentists, the lower, *iri-ibeh* which means dentist ('the one from the tooth', 'the one that treats teeth'),[676] and the elite referred to as *uer-iri-ibeh*, Chief of dentists.[677] Several papyri list prescriptions for dental diseases such as periodontal disease, loose teeth, caries and abscesses.

Surgical holes made to drain an abscess under the first molar were found in the mandible of a mummy from the IVth Dynasty (2625-2510 BC).[678]

A loose tooth repaired with a gold wired bridge connected to a neighbouring healthy tooth (two molars), was discovered in a mummy from the same Dynasty at Giza.[679] Artificial teeth that support a maxillary bridge with a silver string were also found in Greco-Roman period. Extraction of the tooth, treatment of the mouth, of the ulcers in gingiva and treatment of temporal maxillary joint dislocation are mentioned in the *Edwin Smith* and *Ebers Papyri*. Caries were not as common as now, but abrasion of teeth was frequent and the cause was the hard bread; the sand involved in manufacturing was very abrasive.

The eleven therapeutics described in the *Ebers Papyrus* were of external application but they had a more magic than healing function. These purulencies as the papyrus called then, were treated ineffectively as teeth fell out anyway.

An example: The cyst found in the mummy of DjedMaatinesankh, priestess of the temple of Amun-Ra at Thebes, from the Greco-Roman period, exposed at the Royal Ontario Museum, was analyzed.[680] Stephanie Holowka, from The Hospital for Sick Children, Canada, made the digital reconstruction of DjedMaatinesankh, tooth by tooth. There was a huge wound, resulting from an abscess caused by a cyst; and thirteen minor abscesses. One of the canines of DjedMaatinesankh was impactated and the other three were missing, possibly due to periodontal disease. Tooth enamel was destroyed by wear, and to a lesser extent, destroyed by caries.

According to Tony Melcher,[681] University of Toronto, once the tooth enamel is worn, the dentine is exposed, and something sweet, hot, or cold could cause discomfort. In the case of DjedMaatinesankh, the damage is extensive, as the dental pulp is exposed to the root in 24 of her 28 teeth. "Once the pulp is exposed" says Melcher, "it is an acute pain, a terrible pain. Anything, even breathing cold air, hurts. Trying to eat would be terrible." The dental pulp becomes exposed and rapidly gets infected, the propagation of this infection through the root channel to the bone probably caused DjedMaatinesankh the formation of many abscesses and a cyst filled with pus. The cyst measures 5 ml of volume, the equivalent to a tea spoon, and involves five of the eight teeth in the superior left maxilla. From the five holes in her mandible, close to the large cyst, one must have been a result of at attempt made by a dentist to treat the abscess.

---

[670] Zink, Kingschl, Wolf, Nerlich, Miller, 2001, 267-269.

[671] It is still not final the conclusion of scholars if it was a pre or post-mortem addition to the dentition.

[672] Fleming, Fishman, O'Connor, Silverman, 1980:74.

[673] In October 2006 there were found, by chance, the tombs of three royal dentists: Iy meri; Kem mesu; Sekhemka: http://news.nationalgeographic.com/news/2006/10/061023-egypt.html

[674] In a private letter to F. Filce Leek, as mentioned by him in his article *The Practice of Dentistry in Ancient Egypt*, Journal of Egyptian Archaeology 53, December 1967, EES, London.

[675] Ruffer, 1921: 314.

[676] Jonckheere, 1958: 99.

[677] Jonckheere, 1958: 100.

---

[678] In 1917 E. A. Hooton did not know that these holes could be natural; the abscess can make its way through the mandible to evacuate pus, and the result, circular cavities, are precise holes; Filler, 1995: 100.

[679] H. Junker, published in 1929, discovered in tomb 984 at Giza, Filer, 1995: 100; Ghaliounghi, 1963: 134.

[680] Jack, 1995:1.

[681] Jack, 1995:4.

Dentists, identified in written hieroglyphic by an elephant fang, ⌐ may have existed in ancient Egypt since c. 2800 BC The *Edwin Smith Papyrus*, c. 2500 BC, more than 1500 years before DjedMaatinesankh was alive, indicates that dentists knew how to use fire to drill for medical purposes. There is a case referenced in this papyrus that describes as an abscess was drained in a patient. Melcher estimates that the dental problems of DjedMaatinesankh could have began in her childhood, maybe at 10 or 12 years of age. It is not known, says Melcher,[682] if the Egyptians learned with their neighbours, the Assyrian how to use cloves (*Syzygium aromaticum*) as treatment for tooth pain.

In the *Papyrus Anastasi* IV (BM 10249, 12.5-13.8), from c. 1202-1196, XIXth Dynasty, probably during the kingdom of Seti II, according to Boyo Ockinga: "an Egyptian officer is moaning at a far work post as one of his colleagues, a scribe, wears a twisted face as disease *wesetet* has developed in his eye and the worm grows in his tooth and this private does not want to leave him. "[683] Many mandibles show evidence of small perforations made by dentist surgeons, indicating draining of abscesses.[684]

3.12. Gastroenterological/hepatic

The ancient Egyptians suffered much from constipation caused by excessive food. In certain sedentary professions as musician, scribe or doorman there are recorded cases of obesity, either in art or in texts:

- A statue of the scribe Mentuhotep at the Louvre Museum, showing a discrete obesity and three adipose layers under hypertrophied breasts;
- A statue of Sebekemsaf; wearing a large tunic showing the same adipose layers under the breasts, n. 5801, at the Kunsthistorischen Museum, Vienna;
- The musicians playing instruments in the tomb of NebAmun (TT 65) copied by Denon showing authentic females breasts in their thorax;
- Khufu's relative (Hemiunu), architect of the Large Pyramid at Giza, presently at the Roemer-und Pelizaeus-Museum, Hildesheim, (1962).

Other diseases caused by excess food were indigestion, caused also by constipation and obesity and also by sun exposure in work after meals, the calculi or stones in kidneys and urine retention, treatable according to the age of the patient. During the pyramids' construction the workmen were given huge quantities of radish (*Raphanus sativus*), garlic (*Allium sativa*) and onion (*Allium cepa*), probably for its anti-inflammatory and diuretic properties. Herodotus has mentioned this in his Book II, Chapter 125:

"There are writings on the pyramid in Egyptian characters indicating how much was spent on radishes and onions and garlic for the workmen; and I am sure that, when he read me the writing, the interpreter said that sixteen hundred talents of silver had been paid."

Only during the 20th century was this accepted in the scientific community when an antibiotic in preparation, *Raphanin*, was extracted from radishes, and *Allicin* and *Allisttin* from garlic and onion. A wise procedure in an overcrowded space … it is known that infectious diseases affecting the immune system will also be debilitating and damaging to the hepatic function.

Some prescriptions for the treatment of hepatic diseases, in the *Ebers Papyrus* are medicines for jaundice and others (*Ebers* 477-479).[685]

Plants treating the hepatic function used in ancient Egypt:

Artemisia absinthium
Absinthe is famous since ancient times, for its medicinal 'virtues', being quoted in the *Ebers Papyrus*.[686] Used correctly and not excessively, an infusion may increase the biliary secretion, facilitating the liver function and, ingested half hour before meals, it can act as an appetite stimulant and aid digestion. Dioscorides confirms its use to expel intestinal worms, a practice known in ancient Egypt.[687]

Cynara scolymus
The artichoke, the name being derived from the Arabic *al kharshuf*, was first grown in Ethiopia, and later on in Egypt, probably by the same Arabs in their odyssey for Iberian Peninsula where they called it *alcahofa*. In the IXth and Xth centuries the Italians called it *carciofa*, from *articiocco* and *articoclos*. In Egypt, is it was represented graphically on tables and in sacrificial shrines;[688] as it stimulates bile function (yellowish/brown fluid manufactured in the liver and stored in the gall bladder facilitating digestion, together with other substances produced in the digestive tract).[689]

---

[682] Jack, 1995:5.
[683] Ockinga, 1996.
[684] Reeves, 1992: 17.

[685] Bardinet, 1995: 320.
[686] Oregon State University, Jackson County Master Gardener Association Southern Oregon Research & Extension Center, http://extension.oregonstate.edu/sorec/mg/herbanrenewal/wormwood.htm
[687] Manniche, 1989: 80.
[688] Swedish Medical Centre, Seattle, Washington, USA: http://www.swedish.org/110799.cfm Colerectic increase bile production. Artichoke leaves were used as diuretic to stimulate kidneys and stimulated the flow of bile in the liver and gall bladder.
[689] In the first half of the 20th century, French scientists began researching the use of artichoke which confirmed the stimulation of kidneys and gall bladder. Italian scientists isolated the compound of artichoke leaf, called cinarine, duplicating the effects. Synthetic cinarine is now used to treat high cholesterol, and dispepsia.
http://www.aurorahealthcare.org/yourhealth/healthgate/getcontent.asp?URLhealthgate="124796.html;
http://bam-international.com/bam/homepage/ag/Produtos__Alcachofra.html

Cannabis sativa

A plant de name *shemshemet*, *šmšmt*, is mentioned in the Pyramid Texts n. 319,[690] at the pyramid of Unas, in some medical papyri[691] and in inscriptions from the New Kingdom.[692] Warren R. Dawson identified this plant as *cannabis* in *Studies in the Egyptian Medical Texts* in 1934.[693]

There are examples of traces of cannabis pollen in Egypt. One of which is from the mummy in Lyon, c. 100,[694] and other three are from soil samples (two from the pre-dynastic period and another from the XIXth Dynasty).[695] We know from Herodotus, c. 450 BC that the Cimmerians (indo-European nomads from Mesopotamia) used *cannabis* in their funerary rituals. Herodotus says that they placed the seeds in burning coal in small tents and then breathed in the smoke. They brought this culture from Asia c. 2300 to 1000 BC into Africa.[696]

It was used in fumigations and medical unguents during all the Pharaonic periods.[697] In the Egyptian medical papyri, there is also information about a plant from which ropes were made and that could be *cannabis*. But there are no records of its action as a narcotic.

The *nepenthe* from Homer,[698] a drug of forgetfulness, was identified by some authors as *cannabis*, but it could have also have referred to a preparation with *Hyoscyamus muticus*, a familiar plant to ancient Egyptians.[699]

Cichorium intybus

Chicory, many times used as a substitute for coffee. Pliny is the best source available to mention two types in ancient Egypt: the wild one and the grown one. Its juice, with rose oil and vinegar, relieves migraines; it was drunk with wine to treat the liver and bladder.[700]

Cumin cyminum

Cumin was indigenous to Egypt. Its seeds, shaped as little grains, are used as a spice in food since antiquity, considered to be a digestive stimulant and effective against flatulence. Cumin was frequently used together with coriander to spice food.[701] Black cumin oil was known in Egypt as a precious medicine. At the moment of the opening of the tomb of Tutankhamun, archaeologists found a bottle of black cumin oil, no doubt to ensure lack of pain in the afterlife. Black cumin oil is a natural medicine that stimulates and reinforces the immune system, enabling possibilities of cure for numerous diseases. Probably endemic to Central Asia, cumin has been used for centuries: Egyptians used it as spice and placed its fruits in tombs, as an offering.

Curcuma longa, Curcuma domestica, Curcuma aromatica

Turmeric. It is a yellowish-orange vegetable, obtained from a plant's root, endemic to India and imported to Egypt. Its name derives from *kurkum*, its Arabic designation. This species with large roots or tuberculae are used as spices, sources of starch and colorants.[702]

It closes open wounds, also used to dye skin and cloth, and also for jaundice treatment.

Foeniculum vulgare

Fennel was frequently used in antiquity as an antidote for snake bite.[703] Egyptians already knew this herb although it has no name in pharaonic records; some prescriptions from the Coptic period include it (powder) for treatment of eye diseases but it was the Greeks and Romans who experimented with its medicinal qualities to help the digestive system and to lose weight[704] as well as in cooking.

Glycyrrhiza glabra

Liquorice. Although much used its name was not found in texts from ancient Egypt. It was used to heal wounds when crushed into powder and chewed to cure peptic ulcers and heartburn. A gentle laxative which expels phlegm, calms down the liver and pancreas and eases respiratory problems (asthma, cough).[705]

Used to treat bronchitis, cough, rough throat and furunculosis, it is still today the most popular medicine

---

[690] Mercer, 1952: http://www.sacred-texts.com/egy/pyt/pyt17.htm

[691] *Papyrus Ramesseum* III, section A, column 26 in Bardinet, 1995: 468; *Berlin Papyrus* 3027 in Bardinet, 1995: 477; *Ebers Papyrus* 618, *Hearst Papyrus* 177 and 188 in Bardinet, 1995: 339, 398-399 and *Ebers Papyrus* 821 in Bardinet, 1995: 449; *Berlin Papyrus* 3038 in Bardinet, 1995: 416, 419; *Chester Beatty Papyrus* VI, 13 in Bardinet, 1995: 457 and n. 24 in Jonckheere, 1947: 30.

[692] TT 85, tomb of Amenamhab, XVIIIth Dynasty, Valley of the Kings, Thebes and TT 50, tomb of Neferhotep, Thebes, end of the XVIIIth Dynasty in Porter and Moss, 1960, Vol. 1: 172, 96.

[693] Dawson, 1934: 44-45.

[694] Girard, Michel and Maley, Jean, *Étude Palynologique* in L. e Mourer, R. (ed), *Autopsie d'une momie égyptienne du Musée de Lyon* in *Nouvelles Archives du Museum d'Histoire Naturelle de Lyon*, 1987, 25 :107.

[695] Emery-Barbier, Aline, *L'Homme et l'Environnement en Égypte durant la Période Prédynastique* in Bottema, S., Entjes-Nieborg, G. e Van Zeist, W. (ed), *Man's Role in the Shaping of the Eastern Mediterranean Landscape*, 1990, Rotterdam : 324 ; Leroy, Suzanne A. G., *Palynological Evidence of Azolia nilotica Dec.* in *Recent Holocene of the Eastern Nile Delta and Paleoenvironment in Vegetation History and Archaeobotany*, vol.1, 1992:49; Leroi-Gourhan, André, *Les Pollens et l'Embaumement* in Balaout, Lionel e Roubet, C. , (ed), *La Momie de Ramsès II : Contribution Scientifique à l'Égyptologie*, *Éditions Recherches sur les Civilisations*, Paris, 1985 :163-165. I have to thank Daniel Jacobs and Terence DuQuesne who are researching *šmšmt*.

[696] Some sectors of Egyptian and Ethiopian Coptic Church believe that «the green sacred herb from the field» in the Bible, (Ezequiel 34:29) and biblical incenses, together with sacred unguents, are extracted from *cannabis*.

[697] Del Casal Aretxabaleta, 2001.

[698] (*ne* = not, *penthos* = grief, sorrow). In Homer's *Odyssey*, Nepenthes pharmakon is a magical potion given to Helen by an Egyptian queen that casts away all sorrow with forgetfulness.

[699] Kabelik, 1995.

[700] Manniche, 1989:88.

[701] Manniche, 1989:97.

[702] Lebling, 2006.

[703] Manniche, 1989: 106.

[704] Manniche, 1989: 105.

[705] Manniche, 1989: 106.

for jaundice, dilated stomach, sickness and vomiting and it acts as a diuretic, expectorant, anti inflammatory and anti-septic. It is also used for treatment of inflammation in the womb, urinary tract and other inflammatory diseases as well as Addison disease and viral hepatitis.[706]

In excess, it can lead to high blood pressure, retain fluids in the body and cause cardiac problems, coughs, bronchitis, and roughness in the throat. It is also used to sweeten several prescriptions. Besides that, it encourages the production of many hormones, as hydrocortisone, of anti-inflammatory action. It treats conjunctivitis, the supra-renal glands, hormonal imbalances, the spleen, the kidneys, diphtheria and tetanus.

Humulus lupulus
Lupulus (hop), is also important to mention as it is used in beer fermentation,[707] and it is referenced in The Book of The Dead, chapter 125, where it is stated the preference of the Egyptians for this drink (as beer came from the eye of Ra). In ancient Egypt beer was very popular as, according to Athenaeus of Naucratis, it was "invented to help those who had nothing to pay for wine". In many artistic and written sources it is stated that Egyptians loved *henqet*, a true national drink, preferred by all. Egyptians also thought that beer had therapeutic purposes and high social ranking women used beer as cosmetics, to make skin fresher and soft.

It is in the *Berlin Papyrus* 3038, paragraph 199, that a famous birth prognosis is found:

"Method to recognize if a woman would bear child or not: (you will put) barley and wheat (in two bags of cloth) into those the woman will urinate everyday; the same quantity of cereal and sand in the two bags. If barley and wheat germinate both, she will bear child. If barley germinates (only) it will be a girl; if wheat germinates (only), it will be a son. If neither germinates, she will not bear child. "

This connotation of wheat with male and barley with female may be explained by the phonetic similarity of names; *'it*, wheat similar to *it*, father; *mut*, mother, sounded many times as *mtut*, cereal. This association is given to us by the Demotic text of the Memphite theology in Erichsen.[708]

Apium petroselinum
Celery, in ancient Egyptian *matt hast*; in Coptic *gat* or *ceginh*; "The essential oil that stimulates appetite (...) appears in some medical prescriptions (Egyptian texts) for stomach pains or to "contract urine. "[709]

Ocimum basilicum
Basil; from a Greek name, *basilikon* (royal), considered a royal herb, [710]endemic to India and grown in the Mediterranean. Grown as a culinary herb or spice; a source for essential oils, aromatizing and an ornamental for gardens. Its' extract has an antioxidant action. Used medically for treatment of migraines, cough, diarrhoea, constipation, anti-parasite as well as treating kidney functions. Anti-spasmodic, it relieves stomach pains, carminative, stimulant and an insect repellent. Its oil, especially when combined with camphor, has anti bacterial properties and is excellent for the heart. Used also as aphrodisiac and to stimulate childbirth.[711]

Billiary calculi

The oldest proof of existence of these calculi was found in an intact gallbladder of a Theban priestess c. 1500 BC, autopsied at the *Royal College of Surgeons* in London, but destroyed in a Second World War bombing.[712]

3.13. Urinary/Renal

Kidneys were abandoned many times in mummified Egyptian bodies maybe because they were hidden in the back, located in the anterior peritoneal cavity and therefore difficult for the embalmer to reach. The same happened with female reproductive organs.[713] As a note: the bag used to protect the penis would also be a protection against infections found in still waters of the Nile.[714] Urinary problems in adults were corrected using suppositories made of olive oil, honey, sweet beer, marine salt, and passion fruit seeds.

Ruffer analyzed some urinary calculi in 1908 but he did not detect diseases or parasite's eggs. In the kidneys from six mummies he had analyzed there were cases in which he found calcified eggs of *Bilhiarzia haematobia*. The methods used were chemical ones and they did not present any doubts to the diagnosis.[715]

3.14. Psychiatric

Several documents identify *schizophrenia*, c. 2000 BC as depression, dementia and 'thought' disturbances. The physical heart, *haty* and the, *ib*, heart-thought had the same 'headquarters' in ancient Egypt. Physical diseases were seen as symptoms of the heart and the uterus, having their origin in the blood vessels or purulent, faecal matters, venom or even demons. There are no records that clearly identify psychiatric diseases.

[706]For viral hepatitis still further research is needed, http://www.nlm.nih.gov/medlineplus/druginfo/natural/patient-licorice.html
[707] Murakami, Darby, Javornik, Pais, Seigner, Lutz, Svoboda, 2006: 66.
[708] Erichsen, 1954: 332, 363 e 382.
[709] Manniche, 1989: 78.
[710] *Basileus (Greek)*=king
[711] Manniche, 1989: 128.
[712] Gordon-Taylor, 2005: 241-251.
[713] Bitschai, Brodny, 1956:3-4.
[714] Bitschai, Brodny, 1956:5-6.
[715] Ruffer, 1910: 16.

3.15. Genetic

Starting with the example of Akhenaten as an example for probable genetic diseases based on procreation between family members; as marriages between relatives were common and they are still common in Arabic countries in the present[716] reflecting the perpetuation of pharaonic custom, it is still risky to affirm it as so.

It is still only speculation that the human remains found at tomb TT55 would probably be the ones from Akhenaten. In art, the shape of his body shows female hips, and an elongated skull and maxilla.[717] Through artistic representations we can see that Akhenaten suffered probably from endocrinopaty[718] with hipogonadism[719] showing adiposity. His facial distortion suggest that this might be the result of a pituitary lesion, possibly a chromophobe adenoma.[720] Even without recent investigation it is certain that his unusual pelvis, the thinness of his bones and the facial and cranial structure support a diagnosis for hipogonadism and pituitary cranial dysplasia.[721] Let us not forget that his mummy has not yet been found, so any medical investigation could clarify these hypothesise.

Paula Terrey[722] has so far identified fourteen pathological disturbances that afflicted Akhenaten. Those include: pathological obesity, acromegaly[723] and pituitary tumour, hydrocephaly and Frolich syndrome. In 1993, in *The Journal for the Society for the Study of Egyptian Antiquities* a new theory is published, Akhenaten would have suffered from Marfan syndrome. This theory was explored much later, in 1996, and with another presentation at the ARCE, 2004. Without tissues to test for Marfan' syndrome it is difficult to state what he did suffer from for sure. This connective tissue disorder results from a defect in the gene fibrillin-1. The author of this presentation used lists of diagnosis' criteria for Marfan' syndrome which are used by doctors at the Stanford University Medical Centre. She analyzes the 33 symptoms comparing them with artistic representations of Akhenaten. She does not consider in her conclusions that this was his illness.

Let us consider then, that after exchanging information with specialists and bearing in mind the knowledge of ancient Egyptians, that these would be the probable illnesses of Akhenaten and let us try to eliminate them. He was not obese, as art represented obese people differently to the way that Akhenaten was portrayed. Acromegaly: a unique genetic disorder would be almost impossible as he presented other characteristics/symptoms that are not carried by this disease. A pituitary gland tumour; as it affects growth and his abnormal shape is represented only as an adult; it is improbable that he suffered from this although there are similar characteristics in his daughters.

Once again there are no tissues to detect cardiac problems, another consequence or characteristic of this Marfan syndrome. The eyes, affected by this syndrome do not give us, through artistic depictions or texts any trace or information of his visual ability. Hydrocephaly, or fluid in the skull. Could that have been drained then perhaps through trepanation? Frolich' syndrome is a congenital disorder, more common in males, the person shows a distended abdomen similar to a swollen raisin and this person will have urinary problems besides cardiac arterial obstructions but, for these reasons, infant mortality is high, however, Akhenaten reached adult age... Adding up a new theory, he may have suffered from cystitis, an inflammatory disease of the bladder caused by germs originating in the intestinal tract; a bacterium known by *Escherichia coli*. Another example of this disease can be seen in the Chief sculptor, Bak, at the Berlin Museum.[724] Why not risk the idea that he may have suffered from several diseases? Until it is possible to analyze the tissue, hairs, nails, bone marrow which contain his DNA, how about a hepatic dysfunction with effects in the thyroid which affects growth?

3.16. Respiratory

Respiratory infections would arise from poor hygiene as many people lived together in small villages such as Deir el-Medina. Also through direct contact with infected waters, desert dust, infected and dead animals, toxic plants and insects; these were the main infectious agents transmitting diseases.[725] Mining and quarrying exposed workers and their families to infections and also military campaigns and battles as well as robberies, disputes and arguments would subject people to trauma. Ruffer analyzed several pieces of lungs from Egyptian mummies, as well as vessels from viscera with traces of pathological adhesions which he stated were signs of pneumonia (bacillus).

One of these diseases was anthracosis, characterized by the presence of coal particles in the walls of pulmonary alveolae, impregnating pulmonary tissue It is easily detected today in mining communities, and it was probably caused in ancient Egypt by smoke from lamps and cooking fires inside closed homes.[726]

---

[716] Al-Gazali, 2006:831-834.

[717] Dawson, 2003: 107-110.

[718] Endocrine glands affections.

[719] It results in arrested growth and arrested sexual development and/or reproductive insufficiency.

[720] Not getting colour easily

[721] Aldred, Sandison, 1962: 293-316.

[722] Presented at ARCE, 2006, *Diagnosing Pharaoh: Did Akhenaten Have Marfan Syndrome?* Pages 85-86 of *abstracts*/programme of the57th Annual Meeting of ARCE, New Jersey, 2006 and personal emails.

[723] An abnormal development of hands, feet and head caused by a hypophysis tumour.

[724] The prominent abdomen shown in this statue may reflect a liver disease; ascites; and/or the presence of *bilharzia*, Ebeid, 1999: 220.

[725] Ebeid, 1999: 351.

[726] Fleming, Fishman, O'Connor, Silverman, 1980: 90.

Chapter 4
Medical-magical prescriptions and used ingredients

The pharmacopoeia of ancient Egypt included all that nature offered; from vegetable to mineral ingredients (some toxic when used for an unlimited time), excrements and human fluids, animal extracts, water from the Nile and dirt. Some Greek doctors emphasized plant properties as medicinal but with magical characteristics, so these giving them superior powers. Herophilus, 335-280 BC, from Chalcedonia (present Turkey)[727] said that drugs are not anything *per se*; if they are not employed correctly by humans, as they are the hands of gods if used with reason and prudence.[728]

The word *Pharmakon* gave origin to pharmac (drug), but it meant either medicine, venom or magic, spell or incantation and also "what casts away disease".[729] Either beneficial or evil as Homer says in his *Iliad* and his Odyssey; IV, where Helen takes knowledge of certain drugs; X, where Circe is known as being rich in venoms; and where Hermes gives the antidote to Ulysses. He talks about Egypt and its many drugs, and its specialist doctors. The drug mentioned in Homer's *Odyssey* is a medicine for pain; something that leads to forgetfulness of pain and sorrow. It shows the change from the Latin *nēpenthes*, from the Greek *nēpenthes* (*pharmakon*) and is referred to as having its origin in Egypt. Literally, it means "the one which pursues sorrow" (*ne* = no, *penthos* = pain, sorrow). In the *Odyssey*, *nēpenthes pharmakon* a magic potion is given to Helen by an Egyptian queen, Polydamna;[730] and it is thought that it would have opium as ingredient. *Pharmakon* changes to *pharmakos*— the venom becomes the one giving it. The *Pharmakopolai* were the sellers of drugs (medicines). Theophrastus separates myth from fact; he does not discount beliefs associated with magical properties but he neglects to consider superstition.

These prescriptions had as ingredients Egyptian endemic plants and others that were imported to Egypt from Middle East, Asia and the rest of Africa. In the *Grundriss der Medizin der alten Ägypter,* there are hieroglyphs referring to pharmacological ingredients of which there are a total of nineteen as illegible; 167 as doubtful and 358 are accepted.

4.1 Ingredients

4.1.1. Vegetable ingredients

It is not the aim of this work to elaborate a list of the Egyptian medicinal flora, once that there are already several editions containing that information, but some plants are mentioned as having specific medicinal properties and the ingredients are described in the medical and magical papyri;[731] (cases of hepatic, gynaecological and ophthalmological diseases, etc.). Besides the flora referred to in chapter 3, gastroenterological/hepatic there are more ingredients referenced in Annex I – Egyptian Flora with medicinal-magical-religious properties.

4.1.2. Animal ingredients

From animals they took horns, fat, teeth, bones, milk, eggs, hair and some organs according to the prescription. The ingredients from animals included bile,[732] liver, brain, urine and excrements. Although not used as medicine *per se* they were mixed into medical-magical potions designed to exorcize evil spirits from human body.

Beekeeping was abundant in ancient Egypt as beeswax and honey was much used; honey – *bit* – was a powerful ingredient in the kitchen, cosmetics and Egyptian pharmacy. The first mention of honey, the oldest in ancient Egypt dates from the first Dynasty when the title of "Sealer of Honey" is conceded.;[733] and the oldest representations of bees in action are from the Old Kingdom, in the temple of Niuserre, c. 2400 BC, so, it is probable that honey would already existed in ancient Egypt. The Egyptians are thought to have been the first to rationalize beekeeping.

Honey prevents bacterial growth; from its *inhibine*; a bee enzyme, propolis (bee pollen-wax), and it was used in the embalming process as well as for conservation purposes. Honey was used as a natural antibiotic and applied on wounds as a base for unguents.

Milk, *irdjet* in ancient Egyptian (cow, goat), was taken, and generally heated, to make medical exam. Human milk was used as it was believed it was crucial to cure (if a woman had given birth to a boy, even better).[734] Human milk containers designed for child nutrition contained about 1/10 litre, an approximated quantity of a session of breastfeed. They usually had lids in the shape of a woman's head, a female body with breasts from where the milk came out and also in the shape of the god Bes, making faces, of course, to cast away demons. The

[727] Ptolemy Project, University of Toronto, http://www.ptolemy.ca/history.htm
[728] Von Staden, 1989: 8, 19, 400
[729] Ghalioungui, 1963: 35.
[730] Arata, 2004: 35.
[731] Wessely, 1931: 19-26.
[732] A very common prescription in Arabic cultures is to apply bile in the eyes and eyelids to treat the leucoma, cataracts and other eye diseases; the parallel with the *Ebers Papyrus* are obvious; Ghalioungui, 1969: 41.
[733] Ransome, 2004: 26.
[734] Bardinet, 1995: 306 (*Ebers Papyrus* 368); 311 (408); 342 (642).

specimens found suggest that these were manufactured during a short period of Egyptian history (from the middle of the kingdom of Tutmes III to Amenhotep II) and they could have even been produced in the same shop.[735]

Eggs were not consumed as common food; they were used in prescriptions and decorative painting: egg, *suhet*

Pig, *rri* was not much used as food as it was considered impure, but it was used as an ingredient in curative mixtures.[736] The *Book of Dreams* from the *Chester Beatty III Papyrus* (BM 10683), which is probably the oldest manual in the interpretation of dreams, says that eating an egg is a sign of losing something.

Fish, *rem* was consumed essentially dried; fish was part of the daily diet of ancient Egyptians, although it was considered impure by some priests.

According to Abir Enany in her thesis on diet and kitchens in ancient Egypt,[737] the *fasakhani* (man preparing fish), had the concern of cleaning and removing all organs and spines from the fish so that it was completely clean may avoid bacteria' propagation before it was consumed. It was not eaten by all people: "But it is not permitted [to priests] to taste fish." says Herodotus.[738]

The construction of kitchens was designed so that they were built in the southern part of the building so that all smoke was driven out by northern winds. Many kitchens were built with draining tanks so that the organic fluids from the animal preparation would be drained out, they had also pits where residue and waste was disposed of.[739]

The species *Lepidotus* was forbidden as it had a connection with the Osiris death myth with reference to his lost phallus in the river, eaten by the fish many times identified with Seth.

There were also a fish goddess, [740]*Hatmehyt*, worshipped in the Delta, at Mendes; also identified with *lepidotus*, a common fish in the Nile. The location known as Oxyrhynchus (also the name of a fish) where a large collection of important papyri was discovered, from Greco Roman and Byzantine periods;[741] has the name *Marymus kannume* a fish found in the Nile next to lake Victoria[742] (sometimes identified with the *lepidotus*).[743] The Ethiopian king Pie, XXVth Dynasty, ruling from 747 BC, did not break bread with fish if sharing his meals. The food offerings to the deceased rarely included fish and during some periods, fish as food was considered an 'outlaw'[744] or 'unlawful.'[745]

Some fish species were considered sacred. "And from fish they also cherished that called *lepidotus* as sacred, and also the eel; and these, they say, are sacred for the Nile"[746] Some fish such as *but* and *shep*, were banished by the Egyptians because of their taste, but there are few restrictions to its consumption. The perch, *Lates niloticus*, the catfish (electrical, *Malopterurus electricus*), the carp (*Ciprinus carpio*) and the eels were especially important. The *tilapia Nilotica*, the fish with an elephant face, the tiger fish (*Hydrocynus forskalii*), the moon fish (*Citharinus latus*) and many others were also eaten.

In an article published in *Harvard Magazine* the author draws attention to the fact that ancient Egyptians treated migraines with electrical discharges from certain fish as catfish: "The Egyptians [took] electric catfish out of the Nile and unbeknownst to them, what they were probably doing was electrically stimulating the tissues to stimulate those touches and pressure fibers."[747] Doctors in ancient Egypt also used these native fish from the Nile with electrical properties to treat joints and therefore reduce pain from arthritis.[748] These fish are represented in murals that suggest medical applications. The Roman doctor Scribonius Largus used a ray (*Torpedo mamorata*), to treat a patient with gout and wrote in the year 46 that migraines and other pains could be cured standing still on shallow waters near these electrical fish.[749] For other medicinal uses of the ray, see Pliny, *Naturalis Historia*. These first inscriptions of the use of electrical fish as therapeutic of pain are found in several Egyptian tombs (?) and are part in several daily scenes represented at Saqqara, c. 2750 BC.

---

[735] Allen, 2005: 34.

[736] Ver subsecções de patologias oncológicas e prescriptions medicinais.

[737] Daily Star Egypt, June 2007: *The significance of kitchens for ancient Egyptians* about Abir Enany's dissertation, http://www.thedailynewsegypt.com/article.aspx?ArticleID=7488

[738] Herodotus, 2003: 110.

[739] *Daily Star Egypt*, June 2007: *The significance of kitchens for ancient Egyptians,* Abir Enany.

[740] In 2005 Mark Lehner's team at the *Giza Plateau Mapping Project* found in a tomb, n. 407, the skeleton of a young lady of probable foreign origin, according to her skull's measures and buried together with her body, an amulet of a goddess, Hatmehyt, wearing a fish on top of her head, http://www.aeraweb.org/spec_hatmehyt.asp

[741] http://163.1.169.40/cgi-bin/library?e=d-000-00---0POxy--00-0-0--0prompt-10---4------0-11-1-en-50---20-about---00031-001-1-0utfZz-8-00&a=d&c=POxy&cl=CL5.1

[742] Fleming, Fishman, O'Connor, Silverman, 1980: 12.

[743] Per-Medjed (OxyrhynShus/el-Bahnasa), a cerca de 190 km do Cairo.

[744] More on fish in ancient Egypt in Simoons, Frederick J., 1994, *Eat Not this Flesh: Food Avoidances from Prehistory to the Present*, University of Wisconsin Press, 256-258.

[745] *The Hieroglyphics of Horapollo*, 1.44, "To denote a thing unlawful, or an abomination, they delineate a Fish, because the feeding upon fish is considered in the sacred rites as abominable, and a pollution: for every fish is an animal that is a desolator [laxative as food?], and a devourer of its own species", http://www.masseiana.org/hiero.htm

[746] Herodotus, 2003: 124.

[747] *Harvard Magazine*, http://www.harvardmagazine.com/on-line/110525.html

[748] http://www.popularmechanics.com/science/health_medicine/1281016 .html in "By implanting electronic circuits and living tissue, surgeons undo the damage caused by stroke, epilepsy and Parkinson's disease."

[749] http://www.newmediaexplorer.org/chris/2004/09/16/bioelectromagnet ic_medicine_the_book.htm under 'Preface to Bioelectric Medicine-A Brief Historical Perspective'

The first Egyptian written work mentioning electric fish dates from the 4th century, in *The Hieroglyphics of Horapollo*.[750] The nutritive properties were emphasised here....

The Hippocratic writings speak of the *Torpedo mamorata* but do not refer to its curative powers. They only prescribe eating this fish, cooked, to someone that is under nourished. [751]

The traditional eels, according to Pliny the Elder, could be dissolved, two of them, in wine, to cure the dependency on alcohol (*taedium vini adfert*).[752] The same author also refers that muddy rivers should be unless they are filled with eels. A note: eel in Latin is *anguilla*. This is important, as in Greco-Roman Egypt the *anguipedis* (eel-legged creature) could be a medical-magical element in curative amulets giving life and protection.[753] The way to eat them was to cut and cook them (eggs separate), roast them, eat as a *pickle* or simply dried. Herodotus says in Chapter 72:

"[1] Otters are found in the river, too, which the Egyptians consider sacred; and they consider sacred that fish, too, which is called the scale-fish, and the eel. These, and the fox-goose among birds, are said to be sacred to the god of the Nile."[754]

The *Harris Papyrus* mentions that the temple of Amun would have, at a certain time, 441,000 whole, middle sized, catfish. There is an inscription about the weight to measure fish portions used at Deir el-Medina.[755] A record shows that a team of fishermen brought fish to every two teams of workmen at Deir el-Medina, one for the left side and another for the right side. Several times fresh fish was delivered to the doorman and all this was recorded by the team scribe. The fish was measured, although quantities vary. According to the ostracon MC25592, the team Chief from the right side received four parts, ten of the workmen received two parts and a half, the scribe kept two parts and eight men had to take only one part and a half...

Fish was highly used in magic for protection. Under the shape of the *adj* fish an amulet is suspended around the neck of a child to cast away 'dangerous deceased'.[756]

4.1.3. Mineral ingredients

The *Ebers Papyrus* contains several mineral ingredients as alabaster, antimony, hematite, lapis lazuli, iron, led, copper, natron, 'statues scrapes' and copper 'green'.[757] Many of the more effective prescriptions contained small doses of toxic minerals, such as copper oxide (Cu_2O), copper sulphate and native copper, being the first metal used by man. The Egyptians also found that adding small quantities of tin (Sn) would improve metal fusion and so they perfected the methods to make bronze; while observing the durability of this material they represented copper with the *ankh*, symbol of eternal life.

Also used as quoted above:

Alabaster, calcite (calcium hydrocarbonate), $CaCo_3$, was used as powder for mixtures of eye treatments.
Led, *Pb*, from the Latin *plumbum*, it is a known metal in all antiquity.
Galena, *mesdemet*, led sulphide (PbS) was used in eye protection.
Granite, *mat*;
Hematite, *dedi*;
Lapis lazuli, *khesbedj*,

Marine salt, ; *hemat*,

Natron, , *hesmen*,

and *imeru*, an unknown substance described in the *Edwin Smith Papyrus* to treat a broken arm, amongst other ingredients.

Arsenic, (As), from the Latin *arsenium*, was used in antiquity for therapeutic purposes and it is now discarded from present treatments. The interest in the use of arsenic trioxide was recently renewed to use in the treatment of patients with *leucemia promiocelítica aguda*. Arsenic (*yellow auripigment*)[758] is known from remote times as some of its components, especially its sulphates. Both Dioscorides and Pliny knew its properties; Celsius Aurelianus and Galen knew about its irritating effects, toxic and corrosive parasite action, as well as its virtues against cough, vocal cords affections and dyspnoea (shortness of air). Arab doctors also used compounds of arsenic to inhale, taken in pills and potions, and also for external applications.

---

[750] http://www.sacred-texts.com/egy/hh/index.htm
[751] Kellaway, 1946: 120-127.
[752] Pliny, *The Natural History*, book 32, Chapter 49, Methods to prevent intoxication. A surmullet stifled in wine; the fish called *rubellio*; or a couple of eels similarly treated; or a grapefish, left to putrefy in wine, all of them, produce an aversion to wine in those who drink thereof. http://www.perseus.tufts.edu/cgi-bin/ptext?doc=Perseus%3Atext%3A1999.02.0137&layout=&loc=32.49#anch1
[753] Veiga, 2008, *A Preliminary Study of MNA E540, a Graeco-Egyptian Gemstone at the National Museum of Archaeology in Lisbon, Portugal*, Current Research in Egyptology 2007, 141-150
[754] Herodotus, 2003.
[755] Cerny, 1937-1938.
[756] Koenig, 1979: 108.

[757] Bryan, 1974: 19-24.
[758] From the Persian meaning yellow pigment, Bentley, Ronald; Chasteen, Thomas G., 2002, Arsenic Curiosa and Humanity, The Chemical Educator 7 (2): 51–60,
http://192.129.24.144/licensed_materials/00897/sbibs/s0007002/spapers/720051rb.pdf

Conclusions

Although Herodotus can be interpreted as being partial in his Histories, book II, (37),[759] we have to agree with his report on Egypt from the 5th century BC: "They are religious beyond measure, more than any other people; and the following are among their customs" but nevertheless say, that this zeal in religious observance was translated many times in health prophylaxis and its results were beneficial.[760]

This research work aims to produce an up-to-date picture of these practices' study either prophylactic or therapeutic, because these practices involved much more than simple prayers, spells and handicraft potions. This culture defended a system that covered all basic needs; in modern societies, new needs are satisfied by technique. In a society where writing was reserved only for some people and words were considered powerful, this characteristic was enhanced when we analyze the dedication that ancient Egyptians showed in their cults, as not all rose to the knowledge and the power of its use.

According to James Breasted in his studies about the *Edwin Smith Papyrus* ,[761] there was real medical knowledge as we understand it today, but no records survived from that, that have been found so far; manuals, encyclopaedias or atlases, so that we can prove the distinction between popular beliefs, paranormal elements or magic, and also confirmed scientific practices. The ancients Egyptians did not undermined their cult to the gods whether they had religious or military changes.

Health concerns were assimilated with mythological situations.[762]

The large theological divisions existing in dominant classes affected nothing regarding personal piety; the domestic shrines, the women's prayers or the medical-magical therapies for prophylactic purposes.[763] When the gods are satisfied, they thought, order was re-established, the Maat, secured. There were several worshipped gods according to popular requests for the treatment of diseases, problems with pregnancy and childbirth, wounds or simply for the protection of crops and blessings to ensure fertility.[764] It is unfortunate that, we have an incomplete record of all the medical practices as we have only some papyri, inscriptions in tombs and temples and reflections of diseases in art depictions. There are no books or medical records *per se*, as Titus

Flavius Clemens wrote (known as Clements of Alexandria) when he was in Egypt c. year 200 BC[765] Ancient Egyptians interpreted the causes of misfortunes as exterior agents and so, magic interceded for cure, defending humans against the gods' will. The magician tried to "convince" the forces to assist in human requests and, as benefits were conceded, the enemy was confronted invoking the presence of divinities.[766] In summary, all ancient Egyptian daily life was filled with appeals to the gods, protection requests and treatments, spells to change the course of events, preparation for the afterlife, building the tomb, decorating it and filling it. The interest in preparing for the afterlife would be, by itself, a way of life and in doing so, the ancient Egyptians glorified death as a passage to something better and this would allow them to take much more advantage of the earthly life. We cannot therefore dissociate the importance of magic in healthcare, once there was not a word for medicine; as health was a holistic concept of: wellbeing, hygiene concerns, material and personal prosperity and having a large family. As it is said in *The Illustrated History of Surgery*, Egyptian medicine was an original mixture of superstition, ceremony and rational thought; nothing was ever done without a prayer to the gods, but always together with active scientific principles.[767] Therefore, and after extensive research, we may conclude that it existed as a scientific knowledge as we know it today; once there were records of medical practices, reliefs showing the existence of probable surgical instruments and names given to diseases, some still impossible to identify with precision. A university-hospital may have existed, probably located next to the temple of Amenhotep III at West Thebes, where the Colossi of Memnon are. This hypothesis may be sustained by the many statues of Sekhmet found at the Karnak excavation sites; at the Colossi excavation site, these statues would have been erected around the sacred lake in a half-moon shape; *isheru*. According to one of the teams at the location, from the Museum de Brooklyn, New York, in the precinct of the temple of Mut there are more than two hundred statues and fragments of statues of Sekhmet.[768] Those could have been placed there, moved from the western bank, to be used in other structures, after the New Kingdom, by Nectanebo I in the

---

[759] Herodotus, 2003: 110.
[760] Frequent depilation, the ablutions undressing the body of bacteria several times in a day, as an example.
[761] Breasted, James Henry, *The Edwin Smith Surgical Papyrus, Volume One: Hieroglyphic transliteration, translation and commentary with eight plates*, University of Chicago, 1930.
[762] Meyer, Smith, 1994: 80.
[763] Still today the cult to pharaonic gods is made at domestic altars in popular Egypt homes, more visible outside the big cities and therefore less exposed to technological evolution and family leisure alternatives.
[764] Imhotep, Sekhmet, Hathor, Taweret, Bes, Osiris.

---

[765] "…hence there are forty-two books of Hermes which are absolutely necessary. Of these, thirty-six, containing all the philosophy of the Egyptians, are learned by the above-mentioned officers: the remaining six, relating to medicine and the constitution of the body, and to its diseases and organs, and to pharmacy and the eyes, and lastly to woman, are learned by the pastophori", *Stromata*, or *Miscellania* from Clemens of Alexandria, *VI, Chapter IV.—The Greeks Drew Many of Their Philosophical Tenets from the Egyptian and Indian Gymnosophists*: 633. Also in Sharpe, 1863: 35.
[766] Borghouts, 1978: ix.
[767] Sir Roy Calne, 2000: 26.
[768] Joint excavation from the Brooklyn Museum and the John Hopkins University, New York,
http://www.brooklynMuseumm.org/features/mut/e
http://digdiary.blogspot.com/e
http://www.jhu.edu/~neareast/egypttoday.html

same temple that associates Mut and Amun. Mut was frequently associated with Sekhmet, a goddess to whom people directed their prayers whether in causes of war or health. The idea of having existed 730 statues of Sekhmet next to the adobe temple ordered by Amenhotep III brings out the possibility of more statues being dug out of these surroundings in a near future. According to Zahi Hawass, Chief of the Supreme Council of Antiquities, to National Geographic on March, 14, 2006: "The reason for this large number of Sekhmet statues may be that Amenhotep III was sick and put statues in the temple to heal him".[769] Another theory, from Peter Brand, an Egyptologist at the University of Memphis, Tennessee, USA, in the same piece of news: "One possibility is that the king dedicated all the statues of this goddess in an effort to stave off the disease. " Amenhotep III would have had some dental problems in his middle age and would have given the order to build the temple to placate Sekhmet's wrath and ask her to cure his illnesses; erecting two statues for each day in the year, one for each part, day/night. The Louvre Museum has ten from the 575 existing specimens. The Metropolitan Museum of Art of New York has six; dozens are still on open air at Luxor and Karnak sites, next to the temple of Mut and on the Colossi of Memnon site too; two in the Berlin Museum and 21 at the Turin Museum (not counting the ones in private collections that are unknown to the general public). Egyptian medical and health knowledge has contributed to later medicine such as the work done by Galen and Hippocrates, amongst others from the Classical period, some of them are quoted in this work as illustrations of Egyptian legacy; and also to Arabic medicine contacting with the West in the century VII.

The ancient Egyptians have left us with an extraordinary and we can now appreciate their artistic, religious, architectonic, scientific and literary magnificence, as the Egyptians were the precursors in medicine and not the Greeks. To what extent are the civilizations from the Near East so far apart from our one, swamped by Mediterranean influences that, in their turn, owe their progresses to the Egyptians, in science and medicine? Are not the pharmaceutical prescriptions synthetic copies of medicinal properties extracted from plants and minerals? Are not cosmetics, perfumery and all alternative medicines based on energy transference, phytotherapy, animal substances, accompanying prayers in certain treatments, as they did in ancient Egypt? It will be through analysis and synthesis of work from what is discovered in Egyptian soil, and its interpretation according to their times, as well as the observation of present and deep Egypt that will enable researchers to understand motivations and practices common to ancient Egyptians, as well as any insights into how they would have lived then. We cannot, at this point, attest that it was only science or only magic; the two were in the same concept assisting prophylaxis and therapeutics; a symbiotic relationship, mutually non-exclusive. "A magic

acts as much as medicine".[770] In ancient Egypt they considered disease as an enemy to avoid and to achieve that it was necessary, in many times, to have external aid. As it is still done today.

[769]http://news.nationalgeographic.com/news/2006/03/0314_060314_egypt.html

[770] Referring to magical Greek papyri, in the characterization made by the editors of *The Greek Magical Papyri in Translation, including the Demotic Spells* compiled by Hans Dieter Betz and quoted by Meyer, Smith, 1994: 19.

Appendix I
Egyptian Flora with medicinal-magical-religious properties

The aim of this appendix is not to give an exhaustive list of the Egyptian flora, it is just presented, summarized into known plants and trees[771] which have medicinal/magical/religious,[772] of importance in ancient Egypt. Basic properties are described and also some major applications.

Aloe vera
Prospero Alpini reports that women from ancient Egypt perfumed their private parts with aloe vera,[773] and that aloe's wood was used to compose treatments for fevers and plagues.[774] Ancient Egyptians called aloe the plant of immortality. Two of the most famous Egyptian queens were fascinated by it; Nefertiti and Cleopatra trusted that *Aloe vera* kept their skin wrinkle free and young by drinking its juice and bathing with it too.

In 1500 BC Egyptians recorded the use of this plant to treat burns, infections and parasites. They drank its juice and used it to preserve putrefacted bodies. Paintings showing a stereotyped plant may represent aloe; they are dated from since c. 4000 BC and they are found at temples and tombs of ancient Egypt. Aloe is native of tropical Africa, where related species are used as antidote to the venom found in wounds.

African hunters rub its gel onto their bodies to reduce perspiration and odours. In ancient Greece scientists considered aloe vera as a universal panacea. C. year 60 remarkable doctors such as Dioscorides and Pliny used this plant to heal wounds, skin abrasions, insect stings, gingiva' bleedings, haemorrhoids, dysentery and also as a purge agent.

Its name comes from the Arabic *alloeh* and the Hebrew *halal*, which means bitter, bitter substance, bitter because of the bitter fluid found inside the leaves of aloe. Vera comes from the Latin *verus*, which means truthful. It relieves migraines, calms down skin eruptions, burns, and ulcers.

Mandrake (*Mandragora officinarum*)
Called by the Arabs *luffâh*, or *beid el-jinn* (devil's eggs). As the majority of *Solanaceae* plants, mandrake contains alkaloids: atropine, hioscine, and others. The plant alone, or boiled down into an alcoholic infusion was used as anaesthesia.[775] Dioscorides speaks about the use of mandrake to produce anaesthesia when patients are burned or cut. Pliny the Elder refers the effect of mandrake's scent as inducing sleep. Galen alludes to its power of stopping feelings and emotions. A pain killer, imported from Palestine in the New Kingdom. Poisonous and narcotic. The whole plant contains strong alkaloids: hiosciamine, scopolamine, norhiosciamine, mandragorine and atropine; the drink resulting from its maceration (from the root) is thought to be aphrodisiac.[776] Many erotic references to this plant can be found in love poems from ancient Egypt.[777]

Camphor (*Cinnamomun camphour*)
Endemic to East Asia, especially from the island of Formosa, Japan and Meridional China. An insect repellent, used in soap to disguise the smell of certain ingredients, a cerebral and cardiovascular stimulant and an anti-parasitic (gastrointestinal action). Camphor is a secondary metabolite, which in plants, has the effect of inhibiting growth and development of neighbouring plants. It reduces fevers, calms down gingiva when inflamed and is also a sedative for epilepsy. It treats contusions, muscular pain, and rheumatism.

Cardamomo (*Cardamomum letarria*)
A plant belonging to the family of *cingiberaceas,* a perennial bush identical to ginger. It grows naturally in Sri Lanka and Malabar shores, at an altitude of between 500 to 1000 metres. The fruit is harvested, small capsules which contain from 5 to 9 spherical seeds of a greenish colour. For this reason it is the third most expensive species to obtain after saffron and vanilla. It is used in the manufacture of spiced bread and curry compositions. The Arabs put cardamom into their coffee as a sign of hospitality. It also calms down flatulence, works as an anti-asthmatic, eases breathing, epilepsy, treats women's diseases and paralysis.

Cucumber (*Colocynthus citrullus*)
Endemic to India, it has been grown since antiquity in Asia, Africa and Europe. From its large quantity of water it helps to control body temperature and organic processes, offering nutrients to cells and eliminating waste. Good for muscles and skin. It acts upon acne, arthritis, renal disturbances, eczema, fever, excess weight, high or low pressure, hair loss and fluid retention. For its vitamin A presence it acts upon night blindness, dry skin, fatigue, loss of smell and appetite. Through vitamin E it has action upon cell disrupture and red blood cells, muscular fatigue and cuts out excessive deposits of fat in the muscles. Through potassium it acts upon cardiac arrhythmia, intoxicated kidneys, high blood pressure and general body fatigue. It also acts upon the uric acid, renal

---

[771] List of species of fruits and vegetables from Egypt at the digital library of the University College of London:
http://www.digitalegypt.ucl.ac.uk/foodproduction/fruits.html
[772] Wessely, 1931:19-26.
[773] Alpin, 2007: 294;
[774] Alpin, 2007: 356; 429; 433; 438
[775] Manniche, 1989: 118.

[776] Del Casal Aretxabaleta, 2001.
[777] Fox, 1997:126.

and bladder calculi, gout, rheumatisms, chronic constipation and increases diuresis, works upon the stomach, liver and ulcers. Its juice fights skin impurities and it also stimulates appetite and acts as a freshener. It also reduces the sugar present in blood, controlling diabetes.

Black pepper (*Piper nigrum*)
Scientists examining the mummy of Ramesses II found traces of this pepper lodged in his nostrils and abdomen.[778]

Anise (*Anethum graveolens*)
Calms down flatulence, relieves dyspepsia, works as a laxative and diuretic. A plant which fights stomach and intestine gases and colic also enabling digestive action using the seeds in an infusion, also used in a mixture for migraines. Some anise leaves and flowers were found in the mummy of Amenhotep II. It also stimulates the milk production in lactating women. Its oil, made from its seeds, can be used to rub on the head to kill lice infestations. The same oil can be used to rub the abdomen and calm colic.

Fenugreek (*Trigonella foenum-graecum*)
It helps respiratory disorders, cleaning the stomach, calming the liver and the pancreas, reducing swellings. As a transdermal plaster it helps to treat eye cataracts. In ancient Egypt, fenugreek was used for embalming too. The Romans grew it to feed their cattle and horses; its name comes from the Latin *foenum-grecum* which means Greek hay.

Frankincense (*Boswellia sacra*)
Used to treat throat and larynx infections that bleed, phlegm, asthma, and calming vomitting. To obtain frankincense, a long longitudinal incision is made on the tree and the juice-like-milk leaks and the cut is increased. In three months the resin acquires consistency, turning into a yellow colour. It is then scraped into baskets from the tree and even the part already out of the incision, of inferior quality, is used. It is grown in the southern Arabia coast in Dhofar area,[779] where it is collected by the Bedouin. Its main application is the manufacture of incense. The inhalation of the melted stem relieves both bronchitis and laryngitis. The *kohl*, with which the Egyptians painted their eyes,[780] is made of melted frankincense (the charred remains of the burnt frankincense was ground into a black powder), and/or other resins, also used as depilation agent, and from frankincense a paste is made with other herbs to perfume the hands In colder weather times, Egyptians warmed their bedrooms with a fire where they burned incense, frankincense, benzene and aloe wood also. The word *incense* means originally the aroma given by the smoke of any odourific substance when burned.

Garlic (*Allium sativum*)
This has excellent natural anti-inflammatory properties. It gives vitality, calms down digestion, flatulence, a soft laxative, shrinks haemorrhoids, relieves the body of "spirits" (Herodotus reports that, during the pyramids building the workers were given garlic, onion and radish to chew on, although there is no inscription at the Giza pyramids which confirms this statement). The bulbs after being transformed into a tea have an action against worms and parasites, treating also hypertension, insect stings and casting away snakes and scorpions with its odour, also used in drops for ear pain and atherosclerosis. It is also an antibiotic, tonic, treats colitis and acts as a diuretic. Garlic, besides being food and having anti inflammatory properties was used in Coptic medicine to stimulate the milk production in mothers, treating wounds and also used as laxative together with other ingredients.

Carob (*Ceratonia siliqua*)
Laxative, treating the stomach, an astringent, diuretic, as food; a substitute for coffee, food, sweetener and also animal (cattle).

Pomegranate (*Punica granatum*)
It treats intestinal disorders caused by amoebas (caused frequently by polluted Nile waters), through a substance called tannin; gout, cardiac disorders, women diseases, stomach cramps, mouth washing. It is also another aphrodisiac. A diuretic, vermifuge (anti helmintic) and anti-septic. It treats inflammation in the throat and gums, colic, diarrhoea and intestinal worms.

Celery (*Apium graveolens*)
A laxative, urinary anti-septic, treating the loss of appetite, cleaning blood, easing breathing, fever, enables digestion, reduces swellings, treats arthritis, cleans toxins and acts as a diuretic.

Coriander (*Coriandrum sativum*)
A laxative, aphrodisiac, treating the loss of appetite, easing breathing, helps digestion, regulates absent menstruation, treats colic, stomach aches, migraines, acts as an anti-fungicide, repelling insects. Offered at temples for the king; its seeds were found in tombs such as Tutankhamun's.

Henna (*Lawsonia inermis*)
Astringent treats diarrhoea, and open wounds; also used as dye.

Qat (*Catha edulis*)
A more recent plant used in Arabic Egypt. It would have been imported to Egypt through Ethiopia and used as stimulant.[781] Made as an infusion in water or milk sweetened with honey; more frequently chewed, causes addiction, irritability and loss of sexual power in men if consumed in excess (men are the primary consumers

---

[778] Manniche, 1989: 136.
[779] Southern Oman, on the eastern border of Yemen
[780] Also effective on eye treatments: Györy, 2006: 2.

[781] Cottevieille-Giraudet, 1935:113.

anyway or the sole ones); otherwise noted to relieve fatigue and to reduce appetite.

Lotus (*Nymphaea lotus*)
The water lily, white or blue. The white specimen has round petals and the blue specimen has pointed petals. It blossoms at sunrise. A symbol of immortality, sexuality and health and a sexual stimulant (not scientifically proven).

Peppermint (*Mentha piperita*)
Calms down flatulence, helps digestion, stops vomit, a breath freshener also. Carminative, eupeptic, a stimulant, antiemetic, anti espasmodic and analgesic. It helps to treat fatigue in general, digestive problems, colic, flatulence, vomit during pregnancy, any intoxication of gastrointestinal origin, hepatic disorders, palpitations, migraine, asthma, bronchitis, sinusitis and dental pain.

White mustard (*Sinapis alba*)
Induces vomit and relieves pain. According to Pliny, in his *Naturalis Historia,* book 20, chapter 87: "Mustard, from which we mentioned three types, when speaking about garden herbs, is classified by Pythagoras among the main plants for purge; as none is better to penetrate the brain and the nostrils. Grounded with vinegar, it is used as an unguent for snake and scorpion stings and effectively neutralizing the poisonous properties of mushrooms. "

Moringa (*Moringa pterygosperma*)
The oil from this plant is extensively used in ancient Egyptian medicine either by itself or as a means of application for curative medicines.[782]

Onion (*Allium cepa*)
Diuretic, induces perspiration, stops colds, calms sciatic pain, and treats cardiovascular problems. Anti inflammatory, antibiotic, antiviral, sedative. Treats respiratory disorders (colds, flu and cough), eliminates urinary pain, diabetes, migraine, asthma, urinary infection (onion juice); anti-bacterial, against bee stings, lowering sugar levels in blood, relieves high pressure, burns, abscess, digestion, prevents atherosclerosis, constipation, furunculae, chest angina, abrasion, haemorrhoids, hair loss, colic, anti-spasmodic, renal problems, cirrhosis, cosmetic, another aphrodisiac forbidden to priests with celibacy vows. In the pharaonic world it was used in prescriptions to avoid menstruation (*Ebers* 828) and to prevent blood from being "eaten" by a wounded limb (*Ebers* 724). It was also used in mummification, an onion was displayed on the thorax, pelvis or close to the eyes (probably to finish drying out); its use as a snake repellent is also mentioned.

Opium (*Papaver rhoeas*); (*Papaver somniferum*)
There are no records of opium being used as a drug in ancient Egypt in pharaonic times.[783] According to Prosper Alpine,[784] the Egyptians ingested opium and had hangovers. A type of 'wine of Crete' was prepared together with pepper and other ingredients. The seeds were crushed to produce a powder to mix with a drinkable fluid serving as anaesthetic, treating insomnia and migraines, respiratory problems and easing pain.

Castor oil (*Rincinus communis*)
Made from castor beans, this oil was used to cast away cockroaches and mosquitoes, to induce childbirth contractions and also as a lamp oil.[785] It was also used for purges three times a month, drinking it mixed with beer. It was also used as laxative and for migraines.[786] It promotes lactation, dissolves cysts, softens nodules, acts as a cervical analgesic, a topic contraceptive, an anti-inflammatory and calms sore eyes.

Sesame (*Sesamum indicum*)
Treats asthma.

Wheat (*Triticum dicoccon*)
In medicine it was used in bandages. Stimulating hair growth and used in birth prognostics; treating coughs, relieving constipation, used in eye patches, also relieving swollen legs and also to avoid a pregnancy.[787] The *kamut* is a wheat variety endemic to Egypt and Mesopotamia. It was grown there during thousands of years until being replaced by other varieties of wheat with better production results.

Trees

Conifer Abies (*Abies cilicica*)
A tree which is endemic to Syria. Its oil was used to clean infected wounds. The extracted resin is used as anti-septic material and as an embalming fluid.

Egyptian Plum tree *(Cordia myxa)*
Its name comes from the Greek *mucus,* the pulp of its fruit. This bush from western Indies treated diseases of the lungs. Another specimen from the family, *Cordia*

---

[783] About 1450 BCE opium was prized in Egypt for its medicinal applications as stated in the Ebers Papyrus 782 in a prescription for infant colic: Bardinet, 1995: 360-361; Nunn, 1996:153-6, and poppies were cultivated near Alexandria in the Arab period, c. 650, Hobbs, 1998, Brownstein, 1993. Balabanova links the reference of use of poppy seeds in Ebers papyrus, 782 as having social connotation, Balabanova, 1992.
"Not only is the poppy mentioned as a sedative, but the Ebers papyrus contains a prescription for stilling the pain 'which is caused by worms (in the intestines)'", Thorwald, 1962. "Considerable debate exists over the probability of the opium poppy existing in early dynastic Egypt as well as in Assyria. Gabra, 1956, suggested that the word *shepen* refers to poppy and *shepenen* to the opium poppy. These words appear in most medical papyri and in some papyri devoted to magic, notably the Ebers Papyrus." Emboden, 1995.
[784] Alpin, 2007: 333-341; after a long period (1580-1584) in Cairo, he returns to Venice becoming a doctor for the court. His important botanical studies include: *De medicina Aegyptiorum* (1591) and *De plantis Aegypti* (1592), in the latter describing for the first time the medicinal properties of coffee.
[785] Manniche, 1989:142.
[786] Manniche, 1989:143.
[787] Manniche, 1989:153.

---

[782] Manniche, 1989: 122-123.

sinensis grows at the oasis from the Western desert close to the border with Sudan, but it is rare (*Täckholm* 1974). This tree was grown in Egypt and its seeds were found at several archaeological sites. They have the size of a round cherry, pointed at the base, like a cup shape.

Aromatic calamus (*Acorus calamus*)
Less referred in medical papyri, it may have been more abundant as oil to perfume the air. It is used in Islamic medicine as treatment for inflammations in the stomach and liver.

Fig tree *(Ficus carica)*
Figs were much appreciated and peasants had monkeys taught to catch them. Fig liquor was enjoyed and was also used as laxative.

Egyptian Mimosa (*Acacia Nilotica*)
Called *senedjet* by the ancient Egyptians. Its wood was also used to make furniture. It calms diarrhoea and internal bleedings. Its resin, extracted from the tree, was used to treat burns and also as glue to mend broken bones (*Hearst Papyrus* 221), It was also used in eye treatments (*Ebers Papyrus* 415), wounds (*Edwin Smith Papyrus* 46) and dermatological diseases (*Ebers Papyrus* 105), its' seeds cured finger and toe wounds (*Hearst Papyrus* 191, 194), and 'refreshed the vessels' (*Hearst Papyrus* 238, 249). It was also used as an ingredient for treatment of the mysterious *aaa* disease (*Hearst Papyrus* 83).

Palm tree *argun* (*Medemia argun*)
The palm tree produces an edible fruit in the shape of an ellipse, about 4cm long; this tree still exists today in Sudan. It was an ornamental tree in ancient Egypt and its fruits were found in tombs from the Vth Dynasty.[788]

Palm tree (*Phoenix dactylifera*)
This tree has grown in Egypt since pre historical times and its fruits are eaten fresh or dried. The fruits are used to sweeten liquors; a type of wine can be made from dates and its juice used as sweetener. This 'wine' was also used to wash bodies in mummification procedures. The process of fermentation of this drink was similar to wine manufacture as the fruits were pressed and the fluid left to ferment. Dates were also used as currency; as payment such as were other food in antiquity. In medicine its fruits or juice were used in potions, suppositories, unguents and pumices.[789]

Papyrus (*Cyperus papyrus*)
Dried papyrus was used to expand and dry fistulae and to open abscesses for the applications of curative medicines; burnt papyrus acted as cauterizing agent for wounds.[790]

Vineyard (*Vitis vinifera*)

Raisins were used in the kitchen and as medicinal ingredients.[791] Anti-cancerous, anti-tumour, antioxidant, hepatoprotector, vessel protector. Reduces free radicals.

Juniper (*juniperus phoenicea; juniperus drupacea*)
Digestive, calms pains, calms stomach cramps. It is an anti inflammatory plant not to be used by whoever has renal problems, as it can aggravate the disease.

---

[788] Manniche, 1989:119.
[789] Manniche, 1989:133-134.
[790] Evans, 2002.

[791] Janick, 2002
http://www.hort.purdue.edu/newcrop/history/lecture06/lec06.html

Bibliography

5,000 Years of Egyptian Art, The Diploma Galleries, Royal Academy of Art, London, 22 June to 12 August, 1962, The Arts Council, Shenvall Press, London

Abdelgadir, Moawia, 2006, *Clinical and Biochemical Features of Adult Diabetes Mellitus in Sudan, Acta Universitatis Upsaliensis,* Uppsala

Adams, Barbara, 1998, *Egyptian Mummies,* Shire Publications, UK

Aldred, Cyril and A. T. Sandison, 1962, *The Pharaoh Akhenaten: - A Problem in Egyptology and Pathology, Bulletin of the History of Medicine,* Baltimore 36: 293-316

Aldred, Cyril, (Portuguese version by J. D. Garcia Domingues), 1966, *The Egyptians,* Editorial Verbo, Lisboa

Al-Gazali, Lihadh, Hamamy, Hanan, Al-Arrayad, Shaikha, *Genetic disorders in the Arab world,* BMJ 2006; 333:831-834, doi:10.1136/bmj.38982.704931.AE

Allen, James P., 1997, *Coffin Texts Spell* 261 (1.11), *The Context of Scripture, Vol. I, Canonical Compositions from the Biblical World,* Brill, Leiden

Allen, James P., 2005, *The Art of Medicine in Ancient Egypt,* The Metropolitan Museum of Art, Yale University Press, New York

Alpin, Prosper, *La Médecine des Egyptiens 1581-1584,* 2007, Fenoyl, R. de., (translation from Latin to French), Institut Français d'Archéologie Orientale, Voyageurs 21/1, 2eme edition, Le Caire

Ancient Art Gifts from The Norbert Schimmel Collection, 1992, The Metropolitan Museum of Art

Anubis Project, Illness, Health and Socioeconomic Conditions in the ancient Egypt, a multidisciplinary Project, Coordinator Edda Bresciani, 1998-2000

Arata, Luigi, 2004, *Nepenthes and Cannabis in Ancient Greece, Janus Head,* 7, 1, Trivium Publications, Amherst, New York, 34-49

Araújo, Adauto, Ferreira, Luis Fernando, 1997, Paleoparasitology of Schistosomiasis. *Memórias Instituto Oswaldo Cruz,* Vol. 92, 52008-10-05: 717-717, http://www.scielo.br/scielo.php?script=sci_arttext&pid=S0074-02761997000500028&lng=&nrm=iso >

Ascase Puyuelo FJ, Cristóbal Bescos JA, July 2002, *La Catarata del Alcalde,* Archivos de la Sociedad Española de Oftalmología, 77, 7: 403-4

Aufderheide, Arthur C., 2003, *The Scientific Study of Mummies,* Cambridge University Press, Cambridge

Badiola, Isabel Rodríguez, *Apuntes sobre el Papiro Ebers,* 43-56, Instituto de Estudios del Antiguo Egipto, Madrid,

Bagnall, R., Frier, Bruce W., 2006, *The demography of Roman Egypt,* Cambridge University Press, Cambridge

Baines, John, Malek, Jaromir, 1994, *Atlas of Ancient Egypt,* Equinox Books, New York

Balabanova, S., Parsche, S. & Pirsig, W., 1992, First identification of drugs in Egyptian mummies, *Naturwissenschaften,* 79, 358-358.

Baptista, Carolina, Mazzo Martinez, Meneghelli, UG, Bordini, Carlos Alberto, Speciali, José Generaldo, 2003, *Cefaléia no Ancient Egito, Migrâneas cefaléias,* 6, 2: 53-55

Bardinet, Thierry, 2001, *Les Papyrus Médicaux de L'Égypte Pharaonique,* Fayard, Paris

Bibliothèque Interuniversitaire de Médicine et d'Odontologie

Bitschai, J., Brodny, M. Leopold, 1956, *A History of Urology in Egypt,* Riverside Press, Privately printed, Cambridge, Massachusetts

Bongioanni, Alessandro e Croce, Maria Sole, (ed), 2003,

Booth, Abraham, 1831, *A description of the ancient art of embalming practiced by the Egyptians: with an account of the Egyptian mummy, now exhibiting, which is divested of its bandages,* Robinett, London

Borghouts, J. F., 1978, *Ancient Egyptian Magical Texts,* Brill, Leiden

Borghouts, J. F., 1978, *Ancient Egyptian Magical Texts,* Brill, Leiden

Breasted, James Henry, 1922, *The Edwin Smith Papyrus, a preliminary account,* University of Chicago, Chicago

Bremmer, Jan N., 1999, *The Birth of the Term "Magic",* Zeitschrift fur Papyrologie und Epigraphik 126: 1-12

Brier, Bob, Wade, e Ronald S., January 2001, *Surgical procedures during ancient Egyptian mummification,* Chungara (Arica), vol. 33, n.1: 117-123

Brier, Bob, Zimmermann, Michael, 2000, *The Remains of Queen Weret* Chungara (Arica), Vol. 32, no.1: 23-26

Britto, José E. Fernández e Herrera, José A. Castillo, 2005, *Aterosclerosis,* Revista Cubana de Investigaciones Biomedicas, 24: 3

Bromiley, Geoffrey W., 1995, *International Standard Bible Encyclopedia*: K-P, Wm. B. Eerdmans Publishing

Brown, Terry, 2000, *Ancient Egyptian Medical Practices and Rites, Inscriptions, The Newsletter of the friends of the Egypt Centre,* Swansea, 3: 8-9

Brownstein, M. J., 1993, A Brief History of Opiates, Opioid Peptides, and Opioid Receptors. Proceedings of the National Academy of Sciences, 90, 5391-5393.

Bruschi, Fabrizio, Masetti, Massimo, Locci, Maria Teresa, Ciranni, Rosalba, Fornaciari, Gino, 2006, *Cysticercosis in an Egyptian Mummy of the Late Ptolemaic Period American Journal Tropical Medicine Hygiene,* 74: 598-599

Bryan, Cyril P., 1974, *Ancient Egyptian Medicine: The Ebers Papyrus,* Ares Publishers, Chicago

Bryan, Cyril P., 1974, *Ancient Egyptian Medicine: The Papyrus Ebers,* Airs Publishers INC., Chicago

Bucaille, Maurice, 1989, *Mummies of the Pharaohs, Modern Medical Investigations,* St. Martin's Press, New York

Budge, E. A. Wallis, 1895, *The Book of the Dead, The Papyrus of Ani*

Budge, E. A. Wallis, 1898, *The Book of the Dead, The Chapters of Coming Forth by Day, The Egyptian text in hieroglyphic*, Kegan Paul, Trench, Trubner & CO., London

Budge, E. A. Wallis, 1922, *The Oracles of Life by Amen-em-Apt, the Son of Ka-Nekht, Recueil d'études égyptologiques dédiées à la mémoire de Jean-François Champollion à l'occasion du centenaire de la lettre à M. Dacier relative à l'alphabet des hiéroglyphes phonétiques*, E. Champion, Paris, 431-446

Budge, E. A. Wallis, 1994, *Egyptian Religion*, Barnes & Noble Books, New York

Budge, E. A. Wallis, 1996, *The Divine Origin of the Craft of the Herbalist*, Dover Publications, Inc., New York

Budge, Sir E. A. Wallis, 1920, *By Nile and Tigris: A Narrative of Journeys in Egypt and Mesopotamia on Behalf of the British Museum Between the Years 1886 and 1913*, Vol. 1, London, John Murray

Budge, Sir E. A. Wallis, 1994, *Egyptian Religion*, Barnes & Nobles Books, New York

Buikstra, J.E., Baker, B.J., Cook, D.C., 1993, *What Disease Plagues the Ancient Egyptians? A Century of Controversy Considered*, Biological Anthropology and the Study of Ancient Egypt, W, V. Davies and R. Walter, British Museum Press, London

Bushkuhl, Rachel, 2002, *Readings in Magika Hiera: Ancient Greek Magic and Religion, Ch. 5 Pharmacology of Sacred Plants, Herbs, and Roots*, John Scarborough, Ancient Greek Religion, Honors Classical Studies Colloquium, University of Arkansas

Campillo, Domènec, 2001, *Introducción a la paleopatologia*, Bellaterra arqueología, Barcelona

Cartmell, Larry W., Weems, Cheryl, July 2001, *Overview of Hair Analysis: A Report of Hair Analysis from Dakhleh Oasis, Egypt*, Chungara (Arica), 33, 2: 289-292

Cerný, Jaroslav, 1937-1938, *Deux noms de poissons du Nouvel Empire*, BIFAO 37: 35

Cesarani, Federico, Martina, Maria Cristina, Ferraris, Andrea, Grilletto, Renato, Boano, Rosa, Marochetti, Elisa Fiore, Donadoni, Anna Maria, Gandini, Giovanni, 2003, *Whole-Body Three-Dimensional Multi-detector CT of 13 Egyptian Human Mummies*, American Journal Roentgenology, 180: 597-606

Cesarani, Federico, Martina, Maria Cristina, Grilletto, Renato, Boano, Rosa, Roveri, Anna Maria Donadoni, Capussotto, Valter, Giuliano, Andrea, Celia, Maurizio, Gandini, Giovanni, 2004, *Facial Reconstruction of a Wrapped Egyptian Mummy Using MDCT*, American Journal Roentgenology, 183: 755-758

Chassinat, Émile, 1921, *Un papyrus médical copte, Mémoires publiés par les membres de l'Institut français d'archéologie orientale du Caire* 32, IFAO, Le Caire

Cockburn, Aidan, Edited by, Eve Cockburn and Theodore A. Reyman, 1998, *Mummies, Disease & Ancient Cultures*, 2, Cambridge University Press

Colombini, Maria Perla, Modugno, Francesca, Silvano, Flora, Onor, Massimo, 2000, *Characterization of the Balm of an Egyptian Mummy from the Seventh Century B.C.* , Studies in Conservation, Vol. 45, 1: 19-29

Cottevieille-Giraudet, Rémy, 1935, *Le Catha edulis fut-il connu des Égyptiens?*, BIFAO 35: 99-113

Cuenca-Estrella, Manuel, Barba, Raquel, 2004, *La Medicina en el Antiguo Egipto*, Alterabán Ediciones, Madrid

Currie, Katie, April 2006, *Sections of mummy – Histological Investigation of Ancient Egyptian Remains*, The Biomedical Scientist: 328-331

Daglio, Cristiano, 2005, *La Medicina dei Faraoni, Malattie, ricette e superstizioni dalla farmacopea egizia*, Ananke, Torino

Dasen, Veronique, 1988, *Dwarfism in Egypt and Classical Antiquity: Iconography and Medical History, Medical History*, 32: 253-276

David, A. Rosalie, 1982, *The Ancient Egyptians*, Routledge & Kegan Paul, London

David, A. Rosalie, 2001, *Benefits and Disadvantages of some Conservation Treatments for Egyptian Mummies*, Chungara (Arica), Vol.33: 113-115

David, A. Rosalie, *5000 Years of Schistosomiasis in Egypt*, Chungara (Arica), 2000, vol.32, 1: 133-135

David, Rosalie, 2002, *Religion and Magic in Ancient Egypt*, Penguin Books

David, Rosalie, 2008, *Egyptian Mummies and Modern Science*, Cambridge University Press

David, Rosalie, Archbold, Rick, 2000, *Conversations with Mummies New Light on the Ancient Egyptians*, Harper Collins, London

David, Rosalie, Tapp, Edmund, 1993, *The Mummy's Tale, The Scientific and Medical Investigation of Natsef-Amun, Priest in the Temple at Karnak*, St. Martin's Press, New York

Davis, A., 2000, The Professor Gerald Webbe Memorial lecture: Global control of schistosomiasis, Meeting London School of Hygiene and Tropical Medicine Meeting at Keppel Street London, 12 April 2000, *Transactions of the Royal Society of Tropical Medicine and Hygiene*, Vol. 94, 6, November-December 2000: 609-615

Dawson, Warren R., 2003, *Magician and Leech*, Kessinger Publishing, Whitefish, Montana, USA

Del Casal Aretxabaleta, María Begoña, January 2001, *Plantas para la eternidad*, Chungara (Arica), 33, 1: 161-168,

Della Monica, Madeleine, 1980, *La Classe Ouvrière sous les Pharaons. Étude du Village de Deir el-Medineh*, Librairie D'Amérique et D'Orient, Paris

Denon, Dominique Vivant, 2004, *Viagem ao Baixo e Alto Egypt*, Publicações Europa-América, Lisboa

Derchain, Philippe, 1959, *Le Papyrus Salt 825 (B.M.10051) et la cosmologie égyptienne*, BIFAO 58: 73-80

Desroches-Noblecourt, Christiane, 1967, Commissaire Général de l'Exposition *Toutankhamun et son temps*, Petit Palais, Ministère d'État Affaires Culturelles, Ville de Paris

DuQuesne, Terence, 2002, *La déification des parties du corps, correspondances magiques et identification avec les dieux dans l'Égypte ancienne, La magie en Egypte : à la recherche d'une définition, Actes du Colloque organisé par le Musée du Louvre le 29 et 30 septembre 2000*: 237-272, La documentation française, Paris

DuQuesne, Terence, 2006, *The Osiris-Re Conjunction with Particular Reference to the Book of the Dead*, Thothenbuch-Forschungen, Gesammelte Beiträge des 2. Internationalen Thothenbuch-Symposiums, Bonn, 25 bis 29 September 2005, Harrassowitz Verlag, Wiesbaden

Ebeid, N. I., 1999, *Egyptian Medicine in the Days of the Pharaohs*, The General Egyptian Book Organization, Cairo

Ebeid, N. I., 1999, *Egyptian Medicine in the Days of the Pharaohs*, 96-98, The General Egyptian Book Organization, Cairo

Egypt's Golden Age: The Art of Living in the New Kingdom 1558-1085 B.C., Catalogue of the Exhibition, 1982, Museum of Fine Arts, Boston

Egyptian Art, 2001, The Metropolitan Museum of Art, Winter 1983/84

Emboden, W. A. J., 1995, Art and Artifact as Ethnobotanical Tools in the Ancient Near East with Emphasis on Psychoactive Plants. Dioscorides Press

En Egypte antique, Centre d'information sur la surdité d'Aquitaine, 24 August 2005

Erichsen, Wolja, 1954, *Fragments memphitischer Theologie in demotischer Schrift, Papyrus demotische Berlin 13603*: 332, 363 e 382Mainz, Akademie der Wissenschaften und der Literatur, in Kommission bei F. Steiner, Wiesbaden

Erman, Adolf, 1907, *A Handbook of Egyptian Religion*, Archibald Constable & Co, London

Evans, Elaine A., 2002, *Papyrus: a blessing upon pharaoh*, Frank H. McClung Museum, University of Tennessee, Knoxville, USA,

Faulkner, Raymond O., 2006, *A Concise Dictionary of Middle Egyptian*, Griffith Institute, Oxford

Faulkner, Raymond Oliver, 1972, *The Ancient Egyptian Book of the Dead*, University of Texas Press

Fazzini, Richard A., Roman, James F., Cody, Madeleine E., 2005, *Art for Eternity, Masterworks from Ancient Egypt*, Brooklyn Museum of Art, Scala Publishers, New York

Feldman, Robert P., Goodrich, James T., 1999, The Edwin Smith Surgical Papyrus, Child's Nervous System, Classics in Pediatric Neurosurgery, 6-7, 15, 281-284

Ferrari, Daniela, 1996, *Gli Amuleti Dell' Antico Egitto*, Editrice La Mandragora, Imola

Filer, Joyce, *Disease*, 1994, University of Texas Press, Austin

Finch, J. L., *Prosthesis or Restoration? A Detailed Study of the Left Forearm of Durham Mummy*, 2005, DUROM 1999.32.1, MSc Thesis, University of Manchester

Fisher, Ricardo F. Gonzalez, Shaw, Patricia L. Flowers, 2005, *El Papiro quirúrgico de Edwin Smith, Historia y filosofia de la medicine, Anales Médicos del Asociación Médica del American British Cowdray Hospital*, 50,1:43-48

Fleming, Stuart, Fishman, Bernard, O'Connor, David, Silverman, David, 1980, *The Egyptian Mummy: Secrets and Science*, The University Museum, University of Pennsylvania, Philadelphia

Flinders Petrie, W. M., 1890, *Kahun, Gurob, and Hawara*, The University of Chicago Library, Kegan Paul, Trench, Trubner, and Co., London

Fowden, Garth, 1993, *The Egyptian Hermes, A Historical Approach to the late Pagan Mind*, Princeton University Press, New Jersey

Fox, Michael V., 1997, *Cairo Love Songs* (1.50), (*Deir el-Medineh 1266+Cairo cat.25218; Posener 1972*) *The Context of Scripture, Vol. I, Canonical Compositions from the Biblical World*, Brill

Frazer, James George, 2000, *The Golden Bough, A Study in Magic and Religion*, Ch. 3, 4, 38, 39, 40, 41, 42, 54, New York: MacMillan,1922, New York

Galen, 2003, *Sobre las facultades Del Alma Siguen Los Temperamentos Del Cuerpo*, Libraria Clásica Gredos, Madrid

Gamba, Susanna, Fornaciari, Gino, 2006, *The problem of cancer in antiquity: brief review of 94 cases*,

Gardiner, Alan H, 1955, *The Ramesseum Papyri*, Oxford

Gardiner, Alan, 2005, *Egyptian Grammar; Being an Introduction to the Study of Hieroglyphs*. 3rd ed. Revised, Griffith Institute, Ashmolean Museum, Oxford

Gardiner, Alan, 2005, *Egyptian Grammar; Being an Introduction to the Study of Hieroglyphs*, Griffith Institute, Ashmolean Museum, Oxford

Germond, Philippe, 2005, *The Symbolic World of Egyptian Amulets*, 5 Continents Editions, Milan

Ghalioungui, Paul, 1963, *Magic and Medical Science in Ancient Egypt*, Hodder and Stoughton

Ghalioungui, Paul, 1968, *La notion de maladie dans les textes égyptiens et ses rapports avec la théorie humorale, BIFAO* 66: 37-48

Ghalioungui, Paul, 1968, *La notion de maladie dans les textes égyptiens et ses rapports avec la théorie humorale, BIFAO* 66: 37-48

Ghalioungui, Paul, 1969, *Ancient Egyptian remedies and Medieval Arabic Writers, BIFAO* 68:41-46

Ghalioungui, Paul, 1975, *Les plus anciennes femmes-médecins de l'histoire, BIFAO* 75 :159-164

Giuffra, Valentina, Ciranni, Rosalba, Fornaciari, Gino, 2007, *I tumouri maligni nell'antico Egitto e in Nubia*,

Goedicke, Hans, 1963, *Was magic used in the Harem Conspiracy against Ramesses III? (Papyrus Rollin and Papyrus Lee), Journal of Egyptian Archaeology* 49: 71-92, EES, London

Gonçalves, Francolino J., August 2003, *Antigo Testamento e a Sexualidade (*II), revista do Instituto São Tomás de Hereno, Conwind e Centre Culturel Dominicano de Semana de Teologia em Fátima

Gordon-Taylor Gordon, 2005, *On gallstones and their sufferers*, British Journal of Surgery, 25, 98: 241-251

Goyon, Jean-Claude, 1972, *Rituels Funéraires de L'Ancienne Égypte*, Les Éditions du CERF, Paris

Goyon, Jean-Claude, 1977, *Un phylactère tardif, BIFAO* 77: 45-54

Graber-Bailliard, Marie-Christine, 1998, *Papyrus Médicaux de L'Égypte ancienne : Le Traité des Tumeurs (Papyrus Ebers 857 à 877)*, Kyphi, Bulletin du Cercle Lyonnais D'Egyptologie Victor Loret, Lyon, n° 1 : 9-61

Griffith, F. LL., 1898, *The Petrie Papyri, Hieratic Papyri from Kahun and Gurob*, (ed.), London, Bernard Quaritch

Griffith, Francis Llewellyn e Thompson, Herbert, 1904, *The Demotic Magical Papyrus of London and Leiden*, H. Grevel & Co, London, http://www.sacred-texts.com/egy/dmp/dmp00.htm

Guidotti, Maria Cristina, 2001, *Le Mummie del Museo Egizio di Firenze, Maat, Materiali del Museo Egizio di Firenze*.1, Giunti Gruppo Editoriale, Firenze

Guiffra, Valentina, Fornaciari, Gino, Ciranni, Rosalba, 2006, *A New Case of Ancient Restoration on an Egyptian Mummy, The Journal of Egyptian Archaeology*, Vol. 92: 274-278

Győry, Hedvig, 2006, *La Chirurgie dans l'Égypte ancienne*, presentation for the 40° International Congress of History of Medicine, Budapest

Haggag, M. Younis, 1989, *Herbal Medicine in Egypt*, University of Cairo, Faculty of Pharmacy, Pharmacognosy Department, Cairo

Haigh, Carol, 2000, *Estimating Osteological Health in Ancient Egyptian Bone via Applications of Modern Radiological Technology*, Senior Lecturer in Pain Management in the Department of Acute and Critical Care Nursing at the University of Central Lancashire,

Halioua, Bruno, Zuskind, Bernard, 2005, *Medicine in the Days of the Pharaohs*, Cambridge, Massachusetts, London

Harer, W.B., Jr, 1994, *Peseshkef: the first special-purpose surgical instrument*, Obstetrics & Gynecology, 83: 1053-1055

Harris, James E., Weeks, Kent, R., 1973, *X-Raying The Pharaohs*, Charles Scribner's Sons, USA

Hebron, Caroline, 2000, *Occupational Health in Ancient Egypt, The evidence from artistic representation*, Current Research in Egyptology, BAR International Series, Oxford

Heidi Hoffman, William E. Torres, and Randy D. Ernst, 2002, *Paleoradiology: Advanced CT in the Evaluation of Nine Egyptian Mummies*, RadioGraphics, 22: 377-385

Herodotus, 2003, *The Histories, II*, Penguin Books, London

Hobbs, J. J., 1998, Troubling Fields: The Opium Poppy in Egypt. *Geographical Review, 88,* 64-85.

Honeyli, Filippo, (ed), 2006, *A Grande Historia da Arte, 6. Arte Egipcia*, Publico, Porto

Hornung, Erik, 1999, *The Ancient Egyptian Books of the Afterlife*, translated by the German by David Lorton, Cornell University Press, Ithaca and London

Huffman, Carl A., 1993, *Philolaus of Croton: Pythagorean and Presocratic: a Commentary on the Fragments and Testimonia with Interpretive Essays*, Cambridge University Press

Images from Papyri *fac-similes* (Columbia University, USA)

Irish, Joel D., 2004, *A 5,500-year Old artificial human tooth from Egypt: A Historical Note, The International Journal of Oral & Maxillofacial Implants*, 19: 645-647

Iversen, Erik, 1939, *Papyrus Carlsberg NO. VIII with some remarks on the Egyptian origin of some popular birth prognoses*, Ejnar Munksgaard, Kobenhavn

Jack, Lee-Anne, 1995/96, *The Faces of Djed: A CT-scan of a ROM Mummy Illuminates a Life from Ancient Egypt*, Royal Ontario Museum, Rotunda, 28, 3,

Janick, Jules, 2002, *Ancient Egyptian Agriculture and the Origins of Horticulture*, Department of Horticulture and Landscape Architecture, Purdue University, West Lafayette, Indiana 47907, USA, http://www.hort.purdue.edu/newcrop/history/lecture06/lec06.html

Janot, Francis, 2003, *Odontologie et archéologie égyptienne: une femme cordonnière retrouvée sur la pyramide du roi Pépy Ier à Saqqara, Bulletin de l'Académie Nationale de Chirurgie Dentaire*, 46: 35-42

Jardim Botanico, Universidade de Trás-os-Montes e Alto Douro:

Jofre, Gerardo, Septiembre 2004, *El polvo de momia, Boletín Informativo de AE (BIAE)* Año II, XV,

Jonckheere, F., 1958, *Le Bossu des Musées Royaux D'Art et D'Histoire de Bruxelles, Chronique D'Égypte,* 45 : 25

Jonckheere, Frans, 1947, *Le Papyrus médical Chester Beatty (La médecine égyptienne no 2)*, Editions Fondation Egyptologique Reine Elizabeth, Bruxelles

Jonckheere, Frans, 1958, *Les Médecins de L'Égypte Pharaonique*, Édition de la Fondation Égyptologique Reine Élisabeth, Bruxelles

Justin, Renate G., May 2003, *Physician compensation, past and present*, British Medical Journal, Vol. 3: 276

Kabelik, Jan, 1955, *Hemp as a Medicament, History of the medicinal use of hemp, Acta Universitatis Palackianae Olomucensis*, VI, Prague,

Kakosy, Laszlo, Roccati, Alessandro, 1987, *La Magia in Egitto al Tempi dei Faraoni*, Milan, Rassegna Internazionale Cinematografia, Archeologica, Arte e Natura Libri

Kamal, Hassan, 1967, *Dictionary of Pharaonic Medicine*, The National Publication House

Karenberg, A. e C. Leitz, 2001, *Headache in magical and medical papyri of Ancient Egypt, Cephalagia*, London 21: 911-916

Kellaway P., 1946, *The part played by electric fish in the early history of bioelectricity and electrotherapy*, Bulletin History Medicine 20: 120-127

Kieser, Jules, Dennison, John, Anson, Dimitri, Doyle, Terry e Laing, Raechel, 2004, *Spiral computed tomographic study of a pre-Ptolemaic Egyptian mummy, Anthropological Science* Vol. 112: 91-96

Kloos, Helmut, David, Rosalie, 2002, The Paleoepidemiology of Schistosomiasis in Ancient Egypt, *Human Ecology Review*, 9, 1: 14-29

Koenig, Yvan, 1979, *Un revenant inconvenant? (Papyrus Deir el-Medineh 37)*, BIFAO 79 : 103-119

Koenig, Yvan, sur la direction de, 2002, *La Magie en Égypte : à la recherche d'une définition*, Actes du *colloque organisé par le musée du Louvre les 29 et 30 septembre 2000*, Paris, La documentation Française, Paris

Kousoulis, Panagiotis, June / July 2001, *Nine Measures of Magic Part 1: Heka, its theological aspects and importance to the fabric of the Egyptian cosmos, Ancient Egypt Magazine*, 7

Krombach, J. W., Kampe, S., Keller, C. A. e Wright, P. M., 2004, *Pharaoh Menes' death after an anaphylactic reaction - the end of a myth, Allergy* 59: 1234-1235

Lambelet, Riesterer, 1995, *Egyptian Museum Cairo*, Lehnert & Landrock, Cairo

Lawson, Jack, N., 2007, Divination and Obsessive-Compulsive Disorder: A Problem of Perspective? Part II, *Le Journal des Médecines Cunéiformes*, 9: 23-42

Leach, Bridget, 2006, *A Conservation History of the Ramesseum Papyri*, The Journal of Egyptian Archaeology, Vol. 92: 225-240

Lebling, Robert W., *Natural Remedies of Arabia*, (excerpt), *Al-Turath/Stacey International*, 2006,

Leek, F. Filce, 1972, *The Human Remains from the Tomb of Tut'ankhamūn*, the Griffith Institute, Oxford

Lefebvre, G., 1952, *Tableau des parties du corps humain mentionnées par les Egyptiens, Supplément aux Annales du Service des Antiquités*, Cahier 17, IFAO, Le Caire

Lefebvre, Gustave, 1956, *Essai sur la médicine Égyptienne de l'Époque Pharaonique*, Presses Universitaires de France, Paris

Lefebvre, Gustave, 1958, *Observations sur le papyrus Ramesseum V, BIFAO* 57 :173-182

Leitz, Christian, 1999, *Magical and Medical Papyri of the New King*dom, Cambridge University Press, Cambridge

Leitz, Christian, 1999, *Magical and Medical Papyri of the New Kingdom*, Cambridge University Press, Cambridge

Lenoir, (ed.), September 2005, *Le Monde des religions hors-série, 20 clés pour comprendre les religions de l'Egypte ancienne*

Lewis, Napthali, June 1965, *Exemption of Physicians From Liturgy*, The Bulletin of the American Society of Papyrologists, Vol. 2, n.3: 87-92

Liber Herbarum

Lichtheim, M., 1997, *Instruction of Any* (1.46) *The Context of Scripture, Vol. I, Canonical Compositions from the Biblical World*, Brill, Leiden

Lichtheim, M., 1997, *The Destruction of Mankind* (1.24) *The Context of Scripture, Vol. I, Canonical Compositions from the Biblical World*, Brill, Leiden

Lichtheim, M., 1997, *The Legend of the Possessed Princess ("Bentresh Stela") (1.54) (From Karnak, Louvre C284) The Context of Scripture, Vol. I, Canonical Compositions from the Biblical World*, Brill, Leiden

Lichtheim, M., 2006, *Ancient Egyptian Literature, The Old and Middle Kingdoms*, Vol.1, University of California Press, London

Lichtheim, Miriam, 1980, *Ancient Egyptian Literature: A Book of Readings: Late Period* Vol. III, University of California Press, London

Lichtheim, Miriam, 1997, *The Famine Stela* (1.53) *The Context of Scripture, Vol. I, Canonical Compositions from the Biblical World*, Brill

Lichtheim, Miriam, 2006, *Ancient Egyptian Literature*, Vol. I, University of California Press, London

Lisboa, João Vieira, 1978, *A medicina do Egipto antigo*, separata do Boletim Clínico dos Hospitais Civis de Lisboa, Vol. 38, 1-4:267-289

Lopez Espinosa, José Antonio, May-June 2002, *Una rareza bibliográfica universal: el Papyrus medical de Edwin Smith, ACIMED*, vol.10, 3: 9-10

Loret, Victor, 1887, *La Flore Pharaonique d'après les documents hiéroglyphiques et les spécimens découverts dans les tombes*, Librairie J.B. Baillière & Fils, Paris

Louis, A., Christophe, 1967, *Le ravitaillement en poissons des artisans de la nécropole thébaine à la fin du règne de Ramsès III, BIFAO* 65:177-199

Louvre, Les Antiquités égyptiennes I, Réunion des Musées Nationaux, Alençon

Lucas, Alfred, 1911, *Preservative materials used by the ancient Egyptians in Embalming*, Survey Department paper nº 12, Ministry of Finance, Egypt, Cairo

Magdalena, Manuel Juaneda, 2001, *La Paleopatología en Egipto: pasado y presente*, Amigos de la Egiptología en línea,

Malomo, A. O., Idowu, O. E., Osuagwu, F. C., 2006, Lessons from History: Human Anatomy, from the Origin to the Renaissance, *International Journal of Morphology*, 24 (1): 99-104

Mangado, María Luz, (ed.), 2005, *Vida y Muerte en el Antiguo Egipto. Del Arte Faraónico al Faro de Alejandría, Catálogo de la exposición*, Xacobeo, Caixanova

Manniche, Lise, 1989, *An Ancient Egyptian Herbal*, British Museum Press

Marie-Hélène Marganne e Pierre Koemoth, *Pharmacopoea Aegyptia et Graeco-Aegyptia*

Mark Collier e Stephen Quirke ed., 2004, *The UCL Lahun Papyri: Religious, Literary. Legal, Medical and Mathematical*, BAR International Series 1209, BAR Publishing, Oxford

Marx, Myron, D'Auria, Sue H., March 1986, *CT Examination of eleven Egyptian mummies, RadioGraphics*, 6, 2: 321-330

McDonald, Angela, 2000, *Tall Tails, The Seth Animal Reconsidered*, Current Research in Egyptology, BAR International Series, Oxford

Medical report about the mummy that Joann Fletcher stated to be Nefertiti

Medow, Norman B., February, 15, 2006, *Ancient Egyptian records provide clues to ophthalmic care*, Ophthalmology News,

Mercer, Samuel A. B., 1952, *The Pyramid Texts*, Longmans, Green & CO., New York, London, Toronto

Meyer, Marvin W. e Smith, Richard, 1994, *Ancient Christian Magic, Coptic Texts of Ritual Power*, Princeton University Press, Princeton, New Jersey

Miller, R. L., 1997, *Tetanus after cranial trauma in ancient Egypt, Journal of Neurology, Neurosurgery and Psychiatry*, 63: 758

Moodie, Roy Lee, 1931, *Roentgenologic studies of Egyptian and Peruvian mummies, Field Museum of Natural History, Anthropology Memoirs*, Vol. 3, Chicago

Moorey, P. R. S., 2000, *Ancient Egypt*, Ashmolean Museum, University of Oxford

Morse, D., 1967, *Tuberculosis, Diseases in Antiquity: A Survey of Diseases, Injuries, and Surgery in Early Populations*, A.T. Sandison, D. Brothwell, Charles Thomas, Springfield

Morse, D., Brothwell, D. R., Ucko, P. J., 1964, *Tuberculosis in Ancient Egypt*, American Review of Respiratory Disease 90: 524-41

Mostafa, M. H., Sheweita, S. A., O'Connor, P. J., 1999, *Relationship between Schistosomiasis and Bladder Cancer*, Clinical Microbiology Review, 12: 97-111

Mummies; Mummies and Disease in Egypt, University of Illinois

Mummification Museum, 1997, Luxor, Ministry of Culture, Supreme Council of Antiquities

Murakami, A., Darby, P., Javornik, B., Pais, M. S. S., Seigner, E., Lutz, A., Svoboda, P., *Molecular phylogeny of wild Hops, Humulus lupulus L.*, Heredity 97, 66–74, 2006

Nagy, István, 1999, *Guide to the Egyptian Collection*, Museum of Fine Arts, Budapest

Nerlich, A., Zink, A., 2001, Leben und Krankheit im alten Agypten. *Bayerisches Arzteblatt*, 8, 373-376

Nerlich, Andreas G., Wiest, I., Tubel, J., 1997, *Coronary Arteriosclerosis in a male mummy from ancient Egypt, Journal of Paleopathology*, 9, 2: 83-89

New medical Papyrus from the Louvre,

Newsom, S.W.B., 2005, *The history of infection control: Poliomyelitis part 1: Ancient Egypt to 1950 – a disease uncontrolled, British Journal of Infection Control*, 6, 3: 14-16

Noegel, Scott, 2004, *Scorpion Charms and Hippo Tusks: The Power of "Magic" in Ancient Egypt*, lecture at ARCE Northern California Chapter, Berkeley, California, USA

Nunn, John F., 1996, *Ancient Egyptian Medicine*, University of Oklahoma Press, Red River Books, London

Nunn, John F., 1996, *Ancient Egyptian Medicine*, University of Oklahoma Press, Red River Books, London

O'Neill, John P., (ed.), 2005, *The Metropolitan Museum of Art, Egypt and the Ancient Near East*, The Metropolitan Museum of Art, New York

Ockinga, Boyo, 1996, *Macquarie Theban Tombs Project: TT 148 the Tomb of Amenemope, The Bulletin of the Australian Centre for Egyptology*, 7

Okasha, Ahmed, Okasha, Tarek, 2000, *Notes on mental disorders in Pharaonic Egypt, History of Psychiatry*, xi: 413-424

Oliveira, Ana M. A. G, 2005, *Análogos do psolareno com um núcleo de dibenzofurano, xantona ou carbazole: síntese e aplicacoes*, Resumen, PhD thesis, Sciences, Chemistry, Universidade do Minho: 6-7; 40-44

Pääbo S., 1985, *Molecular cloning of ancient Egyptian mummy DNA, Nature*, 314: 644-645

Pääbo S., 1985, *Preservation of DNA in ancient Egyptian mummies, Journal Archeology Science* 12: 411-417

Pääbo S., 1986, *Molecular genetic investigations of ancient human remains*, Cold Spring Harbour Symposium Quant Biol. 51: 441-446

Pack, Roger, A., 1965, *The Greek and Latin Literary Texts from Greco-Roman Egypt*, The University of Michigan Press, Ann Arbor

Pahor, Ahmés L., Chavda, Swarupsinh V., August 2006, *The Great Pyramid: Workmen and their Health*, presentation for the 40º International Congress of History of Medicine, Budapest

Perraud, Milena, October-November 2006, *Les papyrus médicaux, Toutankhamun magazine*, 29: 41-44

Pestman, P., 1982, *Who were the owners, in the Community of Workmen of the Chester Beatty Papyri?*, R. Demaree and J. Janssen, Gleanings from Deir el-Medina, 155-172, Leiden

Petrie, Flinders W. M., 1890, *Kahun, Gurob and Hawara with twenty-eight plates*, London, Kegan Paul, Trench, Trubner, and Co., London

Petrie, W. M. Flinders, 1994, *Amulets: illustrated by the Egyptian Collection in University College*, Martin Press, London

Pettigrew, Thomas Joseph, 1838, *Account of the examination of the mummy of Pet-maut-ioh-mes: brought from Egypt by the late John Gosset, Esq. and now deposited in the Museum in the island of Jersey/ communicated to the Society of Antiquaries by T. J. Pettigrew*, J.B. Nichols and Son, London

Pinch, Geraldine, 1994, *Magic in Ancient Egypt*, University of Texas Press, Austin

Pliny The Elder, 2004, *Natural History: A Selection*, Penguin Books, London

Plutarco, *Isis e Osiris*, 2001, Ediçōes Fim de Seculo, Lisboa

Podzorski, Patricia V., 1990, *Their Bones Shall not Perish, An examination of Predynastic Human Skeletal Remains from Naga-ed-Der in Egypt*, SIA Publishing

Polish Academy of Arts and Sciences, 2001, *Mummy Results of Interdisciplinary Examination of the Egyptian Mummy of Aset-iri-khet-es from the Archaeological Museum in Cracow*, Cracow

Porter, Bertha, Moss, Rosalind Burney, Ethel W., 1960, *Topographical Bibliography Ancient Egyptian Hieroglyphic Texts, Reliefs and Paintings*, Griffith Institute, Oxford

Pott, P., 1779, *Remarks on that kind of palsy of the lower limbs is frequently found to accompany a curvature of the spine*, London, J. Johnson

Prescott, Philip, 1924, *Egyptian mummies: influence on civilization's development*, The Evening Star and Daily Herald, London, Friday January 25

Pujol, Rosa, 2004, *El perfume en el Antiguo Egypt*, Amigos de la Egiptología,

Quartiellers, D. Rodolfo del Castillo, 1909, *Momificación y Embalsamamiento en tiempo de los faraones*, Revista de Medicine y Cirugía Prácticas, Madrid

Quirke, Stephen and Collier, Mark, edited by, 2004, *The UCL Lahun Papyri: Religious, Literary, Legal,*

Mathematical and Medical, BAR International 1209, BAR Publishing, Oxford

Rabino Massa, Emma, Cerutti, Nicoletta e Marin D. Savoia, A., 2000, *Malaria in Ancient Egypt: Paleoimmunological Investigation on Predynastic Mummified Remains,* Chungara (Arica), Vol.32, no.1: 7-9,

Ramirez B., William, 1970, *Host Specificity of Fig Wasps (Agaonidae), Evolution,* 24: 680-691

Ransome, Hilda M., 1937, 2004, *The Sacred Bee in Ancient Times and Folklore,* Courier Dover: 26

Records of the Past, Series 1 and Series 2, 12 Volumes, 1875-1899, Vol. X, *The Magic Papyrus of the Harris Collection,* translated by François Chabas, http://www.brainfly.net/html/books/rop0161.pdf

Reeves, Carole, 1992, *Egyptian Medicine,* Shire Egyptology 15, British Library Cataloguing, Shire Publications, Buckinghamshire

Ritner, Robert K., 1993, *The Mechanics of Ancient Egyptian Magical Practice,* The Oriental Institute of the University of Chicago, Studies in Ancient Oriental Civilization, n. 54, Chicago

Ritner, Robert K., 1997, *Coffin Texts Spell 157, The Context of Scripture, Vol. I, Canonical Compositions from the Biblical World,* Brill, Leiden

Ritner, Robert K., 1997, *Dream Oracles (1.33) (P. Chester Beatty III, P. BM 10683), The Context of Scripture, Vol. I, Canonical Compositions from the Biblical World,* Brill, Leiden

Ritner, Robert K., 2000, *Innovations and Adaptations in Ancient Egyptian Medicine, JNES* 59, 107-117

Robinson, Peter, 2007, *The Locational Significance of Scatological References in the Coffin Texts,* CRE VII, Oxbow Books, Oxford

Roccati, Alessandro, 2003, *Museo Egizio Torino,* nr.1 Nuova Serie, Itinerari dei Musei, Gallerie, Scavi e Monumenti d'Italia, Libreria dello Stato, Istituto Poligrafico e Zecca Dello Stato, Roma

Rodríguez, Ángel Sánchez, 2003, *Papiros medicos, textos medicos, Papyrus Ebers 128, 188 y 251, Papyrus Edwin Smith 4 y 47, Anatomía y Fisiología,* versão online de *La Literatura en el Egipto Antiguo Breve antología,* Egiptomanía S.L., http://www.Egiptomania.com/literatura/medicos3.htm

Roehrig, Catharine H., 2002, *Life Along the Nile, Three Egyptians of Ancient Thebes,* The Metropolitan Museum of Art

Roveri, Anna Maria Donadoni, 2001, *Museo Egizio,* Barisone Editore, Torino

Royal Ontario Museum, 1913, *Theban ostraca: Edited from the originals, now mainly in the Royal Ontario Museum of Archaeology, Toronto, and the Bodleian Library,* Oxford, http://www.archive.org/download/thebyearstracaedi00royauoft/thebyearstracaedi00royauoft.pdf

Ruffer, M. A., 1910, *Note on the presence of Bilharzia hematobium in Egyptians mummies of the twentieth dynasty (1250 - 1000 BC), British Medical Journal,* 2: 16

Ruffer, Marc Armand, 1921, *Studies in the Paleopathology of Egypt,* edited by Roy L. Moodie, The University of Chicago Press, Chicago

Ruffer, Marc Armand, 1921, *Studies in the Paleopathology of Egypt,* The University of Chicago Press

Russmann, Edna R., 2001, *Eternal Egypt, Masterworks of Ancient Art from the British Museum,* American Federation of Arts, London

Saber Gabra, 1956, *Papaver Species and Opium through the Ages,* Bulletin de l'Institut d'Egypte

Sakula, A., 1983, *Augustus Bozzi Granville (1783-1872): London physician-accoucheur and Italian patriot, Journal of the Royal Society of Medicine,* October, 76, 10: 876–882

Salama N, Hilmy A, 1951, *An ancient Egyptian skull and a mandible showing cysts,* British Dental Journal 90: 17-18

Sales, José das Candeias, 1999, *As Divindades Egipcias, uma chave para a compreensão do Egipto antigo,* Editorial Estampa, Lisboa

Salib, Philip, 1962, *Orthopaedic and traumatic skeletal lesions in ancient Egyptians, The Journal of Bone and Joint Surgery,* 44B, 4: 944-947

Sanchez, Gonzalo M., Siuda, Tamara, , December 2002, *Ebers papyrus Case # 873: A Probable Case of Neurofibromatosis 1,* South Dakota Journal of Medicine, , Sioux Falls, USA Vol. 55, 12: 529-535

Sanchez, Gonzalo Moreno, Burridge, Alwyn Louise, July 2007, Decision making in head injury management in the Edwin Smith Papyrus, *Journal of Neurosurgery,* Vol. 23, 1: 1-9

Sandison, A T, April 1967, *Sir Marc Armand Ruffer (1859-1917) pioneer of palaeopathology, Medical History,* 11(2): 150–156

Sandison, A. T., 1967, *Sir Marc Armand Ruffer (1859-1917) pioneer of Paleopathology, Medical History,* April; 11, 2: 150–156

Santos, M. E., 01 January 2003, *Mumias: de Medicina a Estudos Modernos,* AMORCultural, Informativo do Centre Culturel AMORC, 17: 24-33, Curitiba, Brasil

Santos, M. E., Locks, Martha, 01 January 2000, *Restos Egipcios Mumificados da Coleção do Museu Nacional,* AMORCultural, Informativo do Centro Cultural Amorc, 3: 4-11, Curitiba, Brasil

Schoff, Wilfred H., 1925, review of *Un papyrus medical copte by M. Emile Chassinat,* Journal of the American Oriental Society, 45: 76-82

School of Chemistry, Physics & Earth Sciences Flinders University, Adelaide, Australia

Schwarz, Jean-Claude, 1979, *La médecine dentaire dans l'Égypte Pharaonique,* Bulletin de la Société d'Égyptologie, Genève, 2 : 37-43

Sharp, D.W.A., 2003, *The Penguin Dictionary of Chemistry,* Penguin Books, Longman Group, Ltd, London

Sharpe, Samuel, 1858, *The triple mummy case of Aroeri-Ao, an Egyptian priest, in Dr. Lee's Museum at Hartwell House, Buckinghamshire drawn by Joseph Bonomi and described by Samuel Sharpe,* Longman, Brown, Green, Longmans and Roberts, London

Sharpe, Samuel, 1863, *Egyptian Mythology and Egyptian Christianity, The Religion of Upper Egypt,* J.R. Smith, London

Shaw, Ian e Nicholson, Paul T., 2000, *Ancient Egyptian Materials and Technology*, Cambridge University Press, Cambridge

Shaw, Ian, 2000, *The Oxford History of Ancient Egypt*, Oxford University Press, Oxford

Shokeir, A. A., Hussein, M. I., 1999, *The urology of Pharaonic Egypt, British Journal of Urology*, 84: 755-761

Sigerist, Henry E., 1967, *A History of Medicine, I, Primitive and Archaic Medicine*, New York, Oxford University Press

Sipos, Péter, Gyory, Hedvig, Hagymási, Krisztina, Onderjka, Pál, Blázovics, Anna, 2004, *Special wound healing methods used in ancient Egypt and the Mythological background, World Journal of Surgery*, 28: 211-216

Sir Roy Calne, 2000, *The Illustrated History of Surgery*, Routledge, London

Smith, G. Elliot, 2000, *Service des Antiquités de L'Egypte, Catalogue General Antiquités Egyptiennes du Musée du Caire, ns 61051-61100, The Royal Mummies*, Le Caire, Imprimerie de L'institut Français D'archéologie Orientale, 1912, Duckworth, London

Soriano, Guillermo Calvo, 2003, *La medicina en el antiguo Egipto, Paedaytrica*, 5, 1:44-50,

Spindler, Konrad, Wilfing, Harald, Rastbichler-Zissernig, Elisabeth, Nothdurfter, Hans, 1996, *Human Mummies: A Global Survey of Their Status and the Techniques of Conservation*, Springer

Stern, B., Heron, C., Corr, L., Serpico, M., Bourriau, J., 2003, *Compositional variations in aged and heated pistacia resin found in Late Bronze Age Canaanite Amphoure and Bowls from Amarna, Egypt, Archaeometry*, 45, 3: 457-469

Steuer, Robert O., 1948, *Aetiological Principle of Pyaemia in ancient Egyptian medicine, Supplements to the Bulletin of the History of Medicine*, n°10, Baltimore, The Johns Hopkins Press

Strouhal, Eugen, 1978, *Ancient Egyptian Case of Carcinoma, Bulletin of the New York Academy of Medicine*, second series, New York 54: 290-302

Sullivan, R., 2001, *Deformity – A Modern Western Prejudice with Ancient Origins, Proceedings of the Royal College of Physicians of Edinburgh*, 31: 262-266

Sullivan, Richard, 1995, *A brief Journey into medical care and disease in Ancient Egypt, Journal of the Royal Society of Medicine*, 88: 141-145

Sullivan, Richard, August 1996, *The identity and work of the ancient Egyptian surgeon*, Journal of the Royal Society of Medicine, Vol. 89: 467-473

Szpakowska, Kasia, 2003, *Behind Closed Eyes, Dreams and Nightmares in Ancient Egypt*, The Classical Press of Wales, Swansea

Szpakowska, Kasia, 2006, *Through a Glass Darkly, Magic, dreams and prophecy in ancient Egypt*, The Classical Press of Wales, Swansea

Täckholm, V., 1974, *Students' flora of Egypt*, Cairo University Press, Cairo, Egypt

Taylor, John, H., 2004, *Mummy: the inside story*, The British Museum Press

The British Museum Book of Ancient Egypt, The British Museum Press, London, 2007

The Gods of Ancient Egypt, permanent exhibition in the Kraców Archaeological Museum, Kraców, 2003

The Papyrus Carlsberg Collection, http://webarkiv.hum.ku.dk/cni/papcoll/pap_bibl.html

The Treasures of Ancient Egypt from the Egyptian Museum in Cairo, The Rizzoli Art Guides, Vercelli, New York

Thorwald, J., 1962, *Science and Secrets of Early Medicine: Egypt, Mesopotamia, India, China, Mexico, Peru*, Harcourt.

Thorwald, Jurgen, 1962, *Science and Secrets of Early Medicine, Egypt, Mesopotamia, India, China, Mexico*, Thames & Hudson, London

Toutankhamun et son temps, Petit Palais, Ministère d'État Affaires Culturelles, Ville de Paris, 1967

Trindade Lopes, Maria Helen, 1991, *O Livro dos Mortos do antigo Egipto*, Assírio & Alvim, Lisboa

Tunny, Jennifer Ann, 2001, *The Health of Ptolemy II Philadelphus*, The Bulletin of the American Society of Papyrologists, Vol. 38, Issue: 1-4, 119-134

Tunny, Jennifer Ann, 2001, *The Health of Ptolemy II Philadelphus*, The Bulletin of the American Society of Papyrologists, 38, 1-4: 119-134

University College London, *A caution on reading the Ancient Egyptian writings on health*, 2002, http://www.digitalegypt.ucl.ac.uk/med/healingdraft.htm

University College of London, *Fruit and vegetable species from selected sites*, Murray 2000, Mary Anne Murray, *Cereal production and processing: Ancient Egyptian Materials and Technology*, Paul T. Nicholson, Ian Shaw, Cambridge, 505-536

Vassilika, Eleni, 1999, *Egyptian Art*, Fitzwilliam Museum Handbooks, Cambridge University Press, Cambridge

Von Staden, Heinrich, 1989, *Herophilus: The Art of Medicine in Early Alexandria: Edition, Translation, and Essays*, Cambridge University Press, Cambridge

Waddell, L. A., 1930, *Egyptian civilization, its Sumerian origin and royal chronology; and Sumerian origin of Egyptian hieroglyphs*, Luzac, London

Walker, James H., 1996, *Studies in Ancient Egyptian Anatomical Terminology*, The Australian Center for Egyptology, Studies 4, Aris and Philips, Warminster

Walker, James H., 1996, *Studies in Ancient Egyptian Anatomical Terminology*, The Australian Center for Egyptology: Studies 4, Aris and Philips, England

Wessely, Carolus, 1931, *Synopsis florae magicae, BIFAO* 30: 17-26

Wilcox, Robert A. e Whitham, Emma M., 2003, *The Symbol of Modern Medicine: Why One Snake Is More Than Two, Annals of Internal Medicine*, 138: 673-677

Wilkinson, Sir Gardner, 1847, *Hand-Book for Travellers in Egypt including descriptions of the course of the Nile to the Second Cataract, Alexandria, Cairo, The Pyramids, and Thebes, the Overland transit to India, the Peninsula of Mount Sinai, The Oases, &c.*, being a new edition, corrected and condensed of Modern Egypt and Thebes by London: John Murray,

Albemarle Street; Paris, Galignani; Stassin & Xavier; Malta, Muir,

William Ramirez B., December 1970, *Host Specificity of Fig Wasps (Agaonidae), Evolution,* Vol. 24, 4: 680

Winlock, H. E., 2001, *Materials used at the embalming of king Tut-Ankh-Amun,* Ayer Company Publishers, Inc., North Stratford, reprinted by permission of the Metropolitan Museum of Art de New York

Wiss, J. & Sons, Co, 1948, *A story of shears and scissors. Their origin and growth in the Old World and the New, with particular emphasis on the development of the arts of making and selling fine quality shears and scissors in America, which parallels the first hundred years of J. Wiss & Sons Co., 1848-1948,* Newark, New Jersey quoted at http://inwindrs.about.com/library/inwindrs/blscissors.htm

Ziegler, Christiane, Letellier, Bernadette, Delange, Elisabeth, Pierrat-Bonnefois, Geneviève, Barbotin, Christophe e Étienne, Marc, 1997,

Zimmerman, Michael R., 1979, *Pulmonary and Osseous Tuberculosis in an Egyptian Mummy, Bulletin of the New York Academy of Medicine,* New York 55: 604-608

Zink, Albert R., Haas, Christian J., Reischl, Udo, Szeimies, Ulrike, Nerlich, Andreas G., April 2001, *Molecular analysis of skeletal tuberculosis in an ancient Egyptian population,* Journal of Medical Microbiology, 50: 355-366

Zink, Albert R., Sola, Christophe, Reischl, Udo, Waltraud, Grabner, Rastogi, Nalin, Wolf, Hans, Nerlich, Andreas G., January 2003, *Characterization of Mycobacterium tuberculosis Complex Dnas from Egyptian Mummies by Spoligotyping, Journal of Clinical Microbiology,* 41, 1: 359-367

Zink, Albert, Reischl, U., Wolf, H., Nerlich, Andreas G., Miller, Robert, 2001, *Corynebacterium in Ancient Egypt, Medical History,* 45: 267-272

Zucconi, Laura M., 2007, *Medicine and Religion in Ancient Egypt,* Religion Compass 1/1: 26-37

WWW

2006:
http://www.edfeg.com/index.php?page=ancient_med_inst

Al-Gazali, Lihadh, Hamamy, Hanan, Al-Arrayad, Shaikha, *Genetic disorders in the Arab world,* BMJ 2006; 333:831-834,
doi:10.1136/bmj.38982.704931.AE
http://www.bmj.com/cgi/content/full/333/7573/831

Anubis Project, Illness, Health and Socioeconomic Conditions in the ancient Egypt, a multidisciplinary Project, Coordinator Edda Bresciani, 1998-2000
http://www.egittologia.unipi.it/project.htm

Badiola, Isabel Rodríguez, *Apuntes sobre el Papiro Ebers,* 43-56, Instituto de Estudios del Antiguo Egipto, Madrid,

http://www.institutoestudiosantiguoEgipto.com/Papiro_ebers.htm

Budge, E. A. Wallis, 1895, *The Book of the Dead, The Papyrus of Ani*
http://www.sacred-texts.com/egy/ebod/

Budge, E. A. Wallis, 1898, *The Book of the Dead, The Chapters of Coming Forth by Day, The Egyptian text in hieroglyphic,* Kegan Paul, Trench, Trubner & CO., London
http://www.etana.org/abzu/coretext.pl?RC=14900

Budge, Sir E. A. Wallis, 1920, *By Nile and Tigris: A Narrative of Journeys in Egypt and Mesopotamia on Behalf of the British Museum Between the Years 1886 and 1913,* Vol. 1, London, John Murray
http://fax.libs.uga.edu/DS49xB8x1920/1f/by_nile_and_tigris_v1.pdf

Bulletin of the American Society of Papyrologists
http://quod.lib.umich.edu/b/basp/

Bushkuhl, Rachel, 2002, *Readings in Magika Hiera: Ancient Greek Magic and Religion, Ch. 5 Pharmacology of Sacred Plants, Herbs, and Roots,* John Scarborough, Ancient Greek Religion, Honors Classical Studies Colloquium, University of Arkansas
http://www.uark.edu/campus-resources/dlevine/Magika5.html

Castel, E., *Gran Diccionario de Mitología Egipcia*
http://www.Egyptlogia.com/content/view/462/73/

Castel, Elisa, Gran Diccionario de Mitología Egipcia, 2004
http://www.Egyptlogia.com/content/view/462/73/io

Clemens d'Alexandria, *Stromata,* ou *Miscellania,*
http://www.ccel.org/ccel/schaff/anf02.vi.iv.html

Coptic Medical Society, UK
http://www.copticmedical.com/Medicine%20of%20Pharaohs.htm

Corbella, Jacint, *La medicina en el Antiguo Egipto,*
http://www.egiptologia.com/medicine/medicine/medicine.htm

Digital Hippocrates, A collection of Ancient Medical texts (Aretaios, Celso, Galen, Hippocrates)
http://www.chlt.org/sandbox/dh/

Dominique-Vivant Denon
http://www.culture.gouv.fr/culture/actualites/celebrations2000/vdenon.htm
http://www.egypt.edu/feuilleton/denon/denon01.htm
http://www.napoleonica.org/denon/denon_bio.html

Ebers Papyrus
http://www.hieroglyphen2.de/Wreszinski3/html/blattern_0.html

En Egypte antique, Centre d'information sur la surdité d'Aquitaine, 24 August 2005
http://www.cis.gouv.fr/spip.php?article645

Evans, Elaine A., 2002, *Papyrus: a blessing upon pharaoh,* Frank H. McClung Museum, University of Tennessee, Knoxville, USA,
http://mcclungMuseum.utk.edu/research/reoccpap/reoccpr_pyrs.htm

Frazer, James George, 2000, *The Golden Bough, A Study in Magic and Religion,* Ch. 3, 4, 38, 39, 40, 41, 42, 54, New York: MacMillan,1922, New York
http://www.bartleby.com/196/

Gamba, Susanna, Fornaciari, Gino, 2006, *The problem of cancer in antiquity: brief review of 94 cases*, http://www.paleodisease.it/articoli/Paleodisease/THE%20PROBLEM%20OF%20CANCER%20IN%20ANTIQUITY%20-20BRIEF%20REVIEW%20OF%2094%20CASES.html

Giuffra, Valentina, Ciranni, Rosalba, Fornaciari, Gino, 2007, *I tumouri maligni nell'antico Egitto e in Nubia*, http://www.paleodisease.it/articoli/Paleodisease/I%20TUMOURI%20MALIGNI%20NELL'ANTICO%

Haigh, Carol, 2000, *Estimating Osteological Health in Ancient Egyptian Bone via Applications of Modern Radiological Technology,* Senior Lecturer in Pain Management in the Department of Acute and Critical Care Nursing at the University of Central Lancashire, http://www.assemblage.group.shef.ac.uk/5/haigh.html

Ikram, Salima, *Rock the Oasis*, Archaeology, Archaeological Institute of America, March 2006, http://www.archaeology.org/online/interviews/ikram/

Instituto Oriental de Chicago: http://www-oi.uchicago.edu

Jack, Lee-Anne, 1995/96, *The Faces of Djed: A CT-scan of a ROM Mummy Illuminates a Life from Ancient Egypt*, Royal Ontario Museum, Rotunda, 28, 3, http://www.rom.on.ca/schools/egypt/articles/djed.php

Janick, Jules, 2002, *Ancient Egyptian Agriculture and the Origins of Horticulture*, Department of Horticulture and Landscape Architecture, Purdue University, West Lafayette, Indiana 47907, USA, http://www.hort.purdue.edu/newcrop/history/lecture06/lec06.html

Jardim Botanico, Universidade de Trás-os-Montes e Alto Douro: http://aguiar.hvr.utad.pt/pt/jardins/cons_jbutad_comp.asp

Jofre, Gerardo, Septiembre 2004, *El polvo de momia, Boletín Informativo de AE (BIAE)* Año II, XV, http://www.Egiptologia.com/content/view/565/41/

Kabelik, Jan, 1955, *Hemp as a Medicament, History of the medicinal use of hemp, Acta Universitatis Palackianae Olomucensis*, VI, Prague, http://www.bushka.cz/KabelikEN/history.html

Karolinska Institutet, Sweden: http://www.mic.ki.se/Egypt.html

KNH - Centre for Biomedical Egyptology http://www.ls.manchester.ac.uk/research/Centres/

Kousoulis, Panagiotis, June / July 2001, *Nine Measures of Magic Part 1: Heka, its theological aspects and importance to the fabric of the Egyptian cosmos, Ancient Egypt Magazine,* 7 http://www.ancientegyptmagazine.com/magic_07.htm

Lebling, Robert W., *Natural Remedies of Arabia*, (excerpt), *Al-Turath/Stacey International*, 2006, http://www.saudayramcoworld.com/issue/200605/natural.remedies.of.arabia.htm

Les papyrus médicaux d'Égypte http://www.egypt.edu/egypte/bibliographies/thematiques/textes/papyrusmedicaux/papyrusmedicaux01.htm

Liber Herbarum http://www.liberherbarum.com/Index.htm

Magdalena, Manuel Juaneda, 2001, *La Paleopatología en Egipto: pasado y presente*, Amigos de la Egiptología en línea, http://www.Egyptlogia.com/content/view/358/41/

Marie-Hélène Marganne e Pierre Koemoth, *Pharmacopoea Aegyptia et Graeco-Aegyptia* http://www.ulg.ac.be/facphl/services/cedopal/pages/bibliographies/PHARMEG.htm

Medical report about the mummy that Joann Fletcher stated to be Nefertiti http://www.cbc.ca/disclosure/archives/040113_nef/documents/dna_test.pdf

Medow, Norman B., February, 15, 2006, *Ancient Egyptian records provide clues to ophthalmic care*, Ophthalmology News, http://www.modernmedicine.com/modernmedicine/article/articleDetail.jsp?id=313681&pageID=1&sk=&date=

Merck Manual Online: http://www.merck.com/mmpe/index.html; http://www.manualmerck.net/?url=/Articles/%3Fid%3D210%26cn%3D1747

Mummies; Mummies and Disease in Egypt, University of Illinois http://www.uic.edu/classes/osci/osci590/6_2Mummies%20Mummies%20and%20Disease%20in%20Egypt.htm

Murakami, A., Darby, P., Javornik, B., Pais, M. S. S., Seigner, E., Lutz, A., Svoboda, P., *Molecular phylogeny of wild Hops, Humulus lupulus L., Heredity* 97, 66–74, 2006 http://www.lfl.bayern.de/ipz/hopfen/10585/wk2003.pdf

Musée de l'Histoire de la Médicine de Paris http://www.bium.univ-paris5.fr/musee/

Museum Egipcio e Rosacruz de Curitiba, Brasil http://www.amorc.org.br/Museu.htm

New medical Papyrus from the Louvre, *http://web.culture.fr/culture/actualites/dossiers-presse/papyrus2007/dp-papyrus.pdf*

Noegel, Scott, 2004, *Scorpion Charms and Hippo Tusks: The Power of "Magic" in Ancient Egypt*, lecture at ARCE Northern California Chapter, Berkeley, California, USA http://home.comcast.net/~hebsed/noegel.htm

Pujol, Rosa, 2004, *El perfume en el Antiguo Egypt*, Amigos de la Egiptología, http://www.Egyptlogia.com/content/view/513/45/1/2/

Robert H. Wilkins, MD, Division of Neurosurgery, Duke University Medical Center, Durham, North Carolina: http://www.neurosurgery.org/cyberMuseum/pre20th/ePapyrus.html

Rodríguez, Ángel Sánchez, 2003, *Papiros medicos, textos medicos, Papyrus Ebers 128, 188 y 251, Papyrus Edwin Smith 4 y 47, Anatomía y Fisiología*, versão online de *La Literatura en el Egipto Antiguo Breve antología*, Egiptomanía S.L., http://www.Egiptomania.com/literatura/medicos3.htm

Sameh, M. Arab, Medicine in Ancient Egypt, Arab World Books Articles, 2000: http://www.arabworldbooks.com/articles8c.htm;

Schøyen Collection

http://schoyencollection.com/smallercollect.htm#2634

Sharpe, Samuel, 1863, *Egyptian Mythology and Egyptian Christianity, The Religion of Upper Egypt*, J.R. Smith, London
http://www.sacred-texts.com/egy/emec/index.htm

Tell Tebilla Project, Osteology
http://www.deltasinai.com/delta-11.htm

The Theban Royal Mummy Project
http://members.tripod.com/anubis4_2000/mummypag es1/introduction.htm

Tomb Sennefer TT99
http://www.newton.cam.ac.uk/egypt/tt99/reuse.html

Tomb TT320 http://www.tt320.org/

U.S. National Library of Medicine, Bethesda, Maryland, USA
http://www.ncbi.nlm.nih.gov/betweenz/query.fcgi?C MD=Pager&DB=pmc

University College London, *A caution on reading the Ancient Egyptian writings on health*, 2002, http://www.digitalegypt.ucl.ac.uk/med/healingdraft.ht m

University College of London, *Fruit and vegetable species from selected sites,* Murray 2000, Mary Anne Murray, *Cereal production and processing: Ancient Egyptian Materials and Technology,* Paul T. Nicholson, Ian Shaw, Cambridge, 505-536 http://www.digitalegypt.ucl.ac.uk/foodproduction/frui ts.html

University de Birmingham, UK, Ahmés Labib Pahor:
http://medweb.bham.C.
A..uk/histmed/egypt_pahor.HTML

University de Indiana, USA
http://www.indayna.edu/~ancmed/egypt.Htm

University do Minnesota, USA:
http://www.mnsu.edu/eMuseum/prehistory/egypt/dail ylife/diet_egypt.htm

University Las Vegas, Nevada, USA, *Herbs and Spices II*
http://www.unlv.edu/Faculty/landau/herbsandspices.h tm

Wilkinson, Sir Gardner, 1847, *Hand-Book for Travellers in Egypt including descriptions of the course of the Nile to the Second Cataract, Alexandria, Cairo, The Pyramids, and Thebes, the Overland transit to India, the Peninsula of Mount Sinai, The Oases, &c.*, being a new edition, corrected and condensed of Modern Egypt and Thebes by London: John Murray, Albemarle Street; Paris, Galignani; Stassin & Xavier; Malta, Muir, http://dspace.rice.edu/xml/1911/9190/496/WilEgyp.te i_full.html

Wiss, J. & Sons, Co, 1948, *A story of shears and scissors. Their origin and growth in the Old World and the New, with particular emphasis on the development of the arts of making and selling fine quality shears and scissors in America, which parallels the first hundred years of J. Wiss & Sons Co., 1848-1948*, Newark, New Jersey quoted at
http://inwindrs.about.com/library/inwindrs/blscissors. htm